OXFORD MEDICAL PUBLICATIONS

Acute Medicine Algorithms

Acute Medicine Algorithms

Mervyn Singer
Senior Lecturer in Intensive Care Medicine;
Director, Bloomsbury Institute of Intensive Care Medicine
University College London Medical School

and

Andrew R. Webb
Clinical Director and Consultant Physician,
Department of Intensive Care
University College London Hospitals

OXFORD   NEW YORK   TOKYO
OXFORD UNIVERSITY PRESS
1994

Oxford University Press, Walton Street, Oxford OX2 6DP

Oxford   New York

Athens   Auckland   Bangkok   Bombay
Calcutta   Cape Town   Dar es Salaam   Delhi
Florence   Hong Kong   Istanbul   Karachi
Kuala Lumpur   Madras   Madrid   Melbourne
Mexico City   Nairobi   Paris   Singapore
Taipei   Tokyo   Toronto

and associated companies in
Berlin   Ibadan

Oxford is a trade mark of Oxford University Press

Published in the United States
by Oxford University Press Inc., New York

A catalogue record for this book is available from the British Library

Library of Congress Cataloging in Publication Data
(Data available upon request)

ISBN 0 19 262460 1 (Hbk)
ISBN 0 19 262459 8 (Pbk)

Typeset by AMA Graphics Ltd., Preston

Printed in Great Britain on acid-free paper by
Redwood Books, Trowbridge, Wilts.

Preface

After the success of *Critical Care Algorithms* and, in particular, the value of the didactic, step by step approach in emergency situations, this book represents a collection of algorithms covering the common emergencies faced in acute medicine. With this book we have documented our approach to 66 procedures and situations commonly seen in emergency medicine. Necessary justifications and amplification are given as short notes and bibliography following each algorithm.

This book is aimed at students and doctors in the front line of acute medicine. It details initial management steps but does generally not aim to describe the management of a situation that should, more correctly, be undertaken in a specialist department (such as the ICU).

These algorithms are not intended as a substitute for detailed clinical assessment and thought. They are not necessarily the only way of managing a particular problem; they are simply our approach which has been tried and tested. We would strongly encourage individuals to read and amend them as they see fit for their particular practice or patient. If they can vindicate their changes then the problem has been truly considered!

It should also be remembered that every treatment step carries the risk of associated side effects, particularly the invasive procedures. The possibility of iatrogenic injury must always be borne in mind. The art of medicine lies in the balance of risk and we hope that this book will help in achieving this balance.

We would like to thank the following staff of the University College London Hospitals for their assistance and helpful criticism: Dr S Chandran, Prof L Fine, Prof M Harrison, Dr J McEwan, Dr G Ridgway, Dr M Sampson, Dr S Spiro and Dr A Wilson.

Mervyn Singer
Andrew Webb   March 1994

Contents

Abbreviations   ix

1. General   2
1.1.   Basic resuscitation   2
1.2.   Central venous catheter insertion   4
1.3.   Fluid challenge   6

2. Respiratory   8
2.1.   Upper airway obstruction   8
2.2.   Acute dyspnoea   10
2.3.   Acute respiratory failure   12
2.4.   Acute asthma   14
2.5.   Acute on chronic airflow limitation   16
2.6.   Acute chest infection   18
2.7.   Pneumothorax   22
2.8.   Haemothorax/large pleural effusion   22

3. Cardiovascular   26
3.1.   Cardiac arrest   26
3.2.   Hypotension   30
3.3.   Severe hypertension   34
3.4.   Acute chest pain   36
3.5.   Acute myocardial infarction   38
3.6.   Bradyarrhythmia   42
3.7.   Tachyarrhythmia   42
3.8.   Severe left heart failure   46
3.9.   Pulmonary embolus   50

4. Renal   52
4.1.   Oliguria   52
4.2.   Acute renal failure   52
4.3.   Myoglobinuria/haemoglobinuria/haematuria   56

5. Metabolic   58
5.1.   Hypernatraemia   58
5.2.   Hyponatraemia   62
5.3.   Hyperkalaemia   66
5.4.   Hypokalaemia   66
5.5.   Hypercalcaemia   70
5.6.   Hypocalcaemia   72
5.7.   Hyperthermia   74
5.8.   Hypothermia   78
5.9.   Metabolic acidosis   82
5.10.   Metabolic alkalosis   84

6. Endocrine 86
6.1.   Hyperglycaemic ketoacidosis 86
6.2.   Hyperosmolar hyperglycaemic non-ketotic crisis 86
6.3.   Hypoglycaemia 90
6.4.   Thyrotoxic crisis 92
6.5.   Myxoedema coma 94
6.6.   Hypoadrenal crisis 96
6.7.   Hypopituitary crisis 98

7. Gastrointestinal 100
7.1.   Gastrointestinal bleeding 100
7.2.   Acute variceal haemorrhage 102
7.3.   Acute abdominal pain 104
7.4.   Severe vomiting 106
7.5.   Severe diarrhoea 108
7.6.   Fulminant hepatic failure 110
7.7.   Acute on chronic hepatic failure 110

8. Neurological 114
8.1.   The unconscious patient 114
8.2.   Acute weakness 118
8.3.   Severe headache and facial pain 120
8.4.   Generalized seizures 122
8.5.   Raised intracranial pressure 124
8.6.   Acute cerebrovascular accident 128
8.7.   Meningitis 132
8.8.   Severe myasthenia 136
8.9.   Tetanus 140
8.10.   Brain stem death 142
8.11.   Potential organ donor 144

9. Poisoning 146
9.1.   Acute poisoning 146
9.2.   Paracetamol poisoning 150
9.3.   Salicylate poisoning 152

10. Miscellaneous 154
10.1.   Acute confusional state 154
10.2.   Acute anaemia 156
10.3.   Pyrexia 158
10.4.   Sepsis syndrome 162
10.5.   Anaphylactoid reaction 166

Index 169

Abbreviations

Ab	Antibody	M, C & S	Microscopy, culture and sensitivity
ACTH	Adrenocorticotrophin		
AV	Atrioventricular	MAP	Mean arterial blood pressure
bid	Twice daily	Max.	Maximum
BP	Blood pressure	MI	Myocardial infarction
CNS	Central nervous system	N/G	Nasogastric
CPAP	Continuous positive airways pressure	od	Once daily
		PA	Pulmonary artery
CPK	Creatine phosphokinase	$PaCO_2$	Arterial partial carbon dioxide tension
CPR	Cardiopulmonary resuscitation		
CVA	Cerebrovascular accident	PaO_2	Arterial partial oxygen tension
CVP	Central venous pressure	PAWP	Pulmonary artery wedge pressure
DDAVP	1-deamino-8-D-arginine vasopressin		
		PE	Pulmonary embolus
DIC	Disseminated intravascular coagulation	P/O	By mouth
		P/R	Per rectum
DVT	Deep vein thrombosis	prn	as required
ECG	Electrocardiogram	PT	Prothrombin time
EEG	Electroencephalogram	PTT	Partial thromboplastin time
EMG	Electromyogram	qid	Four times daily
FBC	Full blood count	RBBB	Right bundle branch block
FiO_2	Fractional inspired oxygen concentration	RV	Right ventricular
		S/C	Subcutaneously
FFP	Fresh frozen plasma	SpO_2	Oxygen saturation by pulse oximeter
FVC	Forced vital capacity		
G-I	Gastrointestinal	SvO_2	Mixed venous oxygen saturation
Hb	Haemoglobin		
HbsAg	Hepatitis B surface antigen	T3	Triiodothyronine
HIV	Human immunodeficiency virus	T4	Thyroxine
		TFT	Thyroid function test
ICP	Intracranial pressure	TIA	Transient ischaemic attack
I/M	Intramuscular	tid	Three times daily
I/V	Intravenous	TSH	Thyroid stimulating hormone
JVP	Jugular venous pressure	U&E	Plasma urea and electrolytes
LBBB	Left bundle branch block	VSD	Ventricular septal defect
LV	Left ventricular	WBC	White blood cell count

Key to algorithms

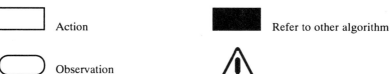

Action

Observation

Refer to other algorithm

Important Note

Acute Medicine Algorithms

1. General

1.1 Basic resuscitation

1. In any severe cardiorespiratory disturbance the order of priority should be:
   - secure the airway
   - maintain respiration (with manual ventilation if necessary)
   - restore the circulation (with cardiac massage if necessary)
   - consider mechanical ventilation
2. CPR may be indicated in cases of severe bradycardia with weak pulse.
3. In the severely hypoxaemic patient oxygen therapy should be in high concentration and at high flow unless there is known chronic CO_2 retention [see algorithm 2.5].
4. In CO_2 retention, failure to restore adequate oxygenation with controlled oxygen therapy requires an increase in oxygen concentration and mechanical ventilation if hypercapnia becomes severe.
5. Initial treatment of hypotension should be with a fluid challenge [see algorithm 1.3] to overcome any hypovolaemia. Life-threatening hypotension may require, in addition, blind treatment with adrenaline (0.05–0.2 mg increments I/V). Invasive monitoring should not be delayed in these cases.
6. Venous access should be secured early during basic resuscitation
   - larger bore cannula if possible, e.g. 14 gauge
   - in haemorrhage two large bore cannulae may be required
   - avoid very small peripheral veins (e.g. on back of hand)
   - use veins in forearm flexures if nowhere else available
   - consider Seldinger access to femoral vein or surgical cut down to peripheral vein in very difficult patient
7. Central venous catheterization is often helpful for continued circulatory management and should be considered once basic resuscitation has been achieved [see algorithm 1.2].

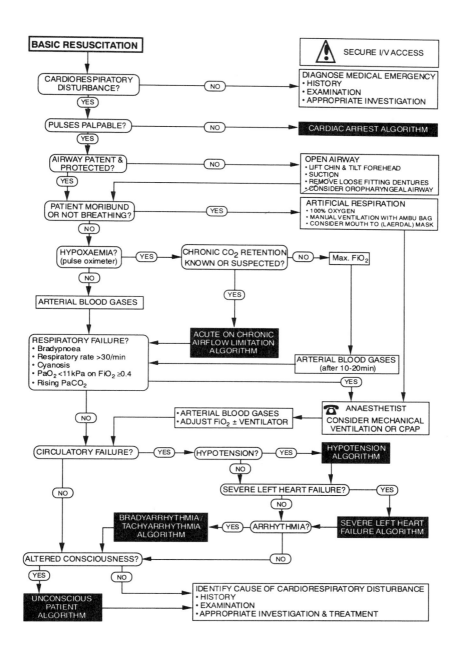

BASIC RESUSCITATION

⚠ SECURE I/V ACCESS

CARDIORESPIRATORY DISTURBANCE? — NO → DIAGNOSE MEDICAL EMERGENCY
• HISTORY
• EXAMINATION
• APPROPRIATE INVESTIGATION

YES

PULSES PALPABLE? — NO → CARDIAC ARREST ALGORITHM

YES

AIRWAY PATENT & PROTECTED? — NO → OPEN AIRWAY
• LIFT CHIN & TILT FOREHEAD
• SUCTION
• REMOVE LOOSE FITTING DENTURES
• CONSIDER OROPHARYNGEAL AIRWAY

YES

PATIENT MORIBUND OR NOT BREATHING? — YES → ARTIFICIAL RESPIRATION
• 100% OXYGEN
• MANUAL VENTILATION WITH AMBU BAG
• CONSIDER MOUTH TO (LAERDAL) MASK

NO

HYPOXAEMIA? (pulse oximeter) — YES → CHRONIC CO_2 RETENTION KNOWN OR SUSPECTED? — NO → Max. FiO_2

NO

ARTERIAL BLOOD GASES

CHRONIC CO_2 RETENTION KNOWN OR SUSPECTED? — YES → ACUTE ON CHRONIC AIRFLOW LIMITATION ALGORITHM

RESPIRATORY FAILURE?
• Bradypnoea
• Respiratory rate >30/min
• Cyanosis
• PaO_2 <11kPa on FiO_2 ≥0.4
• Rising $PaCO_2$

ARTERIAL BLOOD GASES (after 10-20min) — YES

☎ ANAESTHETIST CONSIDER MECHANICAL VENTILATION OR CPAP

NO

• ARTERIAL BLOOD GASES
• ADJUST FiO_2 ± VENTILATOR

CIRCULATORY FAILURE? — YES → HYPOTENSION? — YES → HYPOTENSION ALGORITHM

NO

SEVERE LEFT HEART FAILURE? — YES

NO

BRADYARRHYTHMIA / TACHYARRHYTHMIA ALGORITHM — YES → ARRHYTHMIA? — SEVERE LEFT HEART FAILURE ALGORITHM

NO

ALTERED CONSCIOUSNESS? — NO

YES   NO

UNCONSCIOUS PATIENT ALGORITHM

IDENTIFY CAUSE OF CARDIORESPIRATORY DISTURBANCE
• HISTORY
• EXAMINATION
• APPROPRIATE INVESTIGATION & TREATMENT

1.2 Central venous catheter insertion

1. The Seldinger technique involves locating the vein with a cannula/introducer needle, feeding a guidewire with a flexible 'J' tip through the cannula into the vein, removing the cannula, then introducing the central venous catheter into the vein over the guidewire. A scalpel incision may be needed to enlarge the skin and subcutaneous tissue puncture and a rigid dilator may be used over the guidewire to form a track through the tissues prior to insertion of the central venous catheter.

2. If a severe coagulopathy is present:
   - avoid the subclavian route if possible
   - insertion should be performed by an experienced operator

3. Do not leave in situ a central venous catheter placed in a hurry under non-aseptic conditions (e.g. during a cardiac arrest).

4. Arrhythmias may occur during placement if the guidewire or the catheter passes through the tricuspid valve. These usually settle spontaneously on withdrawing the catheter/wire.

5. The risk of infection with femoral site insertion is no greater provided aseptic insertion technique and proper dressing care is used. A long catheter with the tip within the thorax is required for central venous pressure monitoring.

6. Except in emergencies, correct placement in a central vein/right atrium should usually be confirmed by chest X-ray before administration of drugs/fluid. Good flowback or drawback of blood from the catheter, and/or obtaining a central venous pressure waveform on transducing the catheter are probable though not absolute guarantees of correct placement.

7. The CVP should not be measured during rapid volume infusion. If possible, stop the fluid for 5–10 min to allow equilibration of fluid between intra- and extravascular compartments.

Bibliography

Gray P, Sullivan G, Ostryzniuk P, *et al.* Value of postprocedural chest radiographs in the adult intensive care unit. *Crit Care Med* 1992; **20**: 1513

McGee WT, Ackerman BL, Rouben LR, *et al.* Accurate placement of central venous catheters: a prospective, randomized, multicenter trial. *Crit Care Med* 1993; **21**: 1118

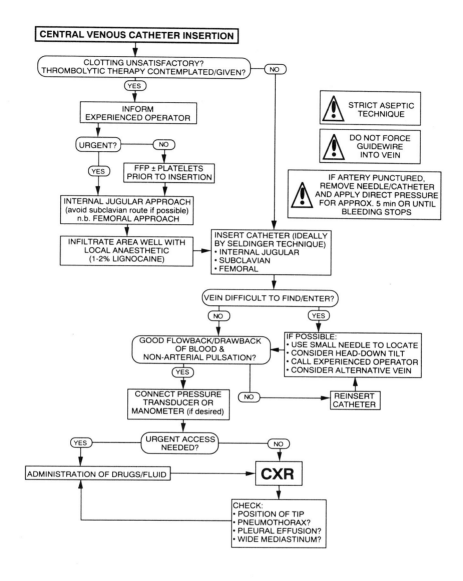

CENTRAL VENOUS CATHETER INSERTION

CLOTTING UNSATISFACTORY?
THROMBOLYTIC THERAPY CONTEMPLATED/GIVEN? — NO

YES

INFORM
EXPERIENCED OPERATOR

URGENT? — NO

YES

FFP ± PLATELETS
PRIOR TO INSERTION

INTERNAL JUGULAR APPROACH
(avoid subclavian route if possible)
n.b. FEMORAL APPROACH

INFILTRATE AREA WELL WITH
LOCAL ANAESTHETIC
(1-2% LIGNOCAINE)

⚠ STRICT ASEPTIC
TECHNIQUE

⚠ DO NOT FORCE
GUIDEWIRE
INTO VEIN

⚠ IF ARTERY PUNCTURED,
REMOVE NEEDLE/CATHETER
AND APPLY DIRECT PRESSURE
FOR APPROX. 5 min OR UNTIL
BLEEDING STOPS

INSERT CATHETER (IDEALLY
BY SELDINGER TECHNIQUE)
• INTERNAL JUGULAR
• SUBCLAVIAN
• FEMORAL

VEIN DIFFICULT TO FIND/ENTER?

NO   YES

GOOD FLOWBACK/DRAWBACK
OF BLOOD &
NON-ARTERIAL PULSATION?

IF POSSIBLE:
• USE SMALL NEEDLE TO LOCATE
• CONSIDER HEAD-DOWN TILT
• CALL EXPERIENCED OPERATOR
• CONSIDER ALTERNATIVE VEIN

YES

CONNECT PRESSURE
TRANSDUCER OR
MANOMETER (if desired)

NO

REINSERT
CATHETER

YES

URGENT ACCESS
NEEDED? — NO

ADMINISTRATION OF DRUGS/FLUID — **CXR**

CHECK:
• POSITION OF TIP
• PNEUMOTHORAX?
• PLEURAL EFFUSION?
• WIDE MEDIASTINUM?

1.3 Fluid challenge

1. Hypovolaemia must be treated urgently to avoid sequelae such as organ failure.
2. Maintain a high index of suspicion for hypovolaemia.
3. Ensure an adequate circulating volume before considering other methods of circulatory support.
4. Repetitive infusion of small aliquots of colloid (or blood) is a safe and convenient method of managing hypovolaemia.
5. Critically ill patients generally require a greater than normal blood volume to maintain adequate circulatory function.

Central venous pressure responses

1. Peripheral vasoconstriction may maintain CVP despite hypovolaemia.
2. The absolute CVP is not a good guide to volume status particularly in chronic cardiac or pulmonary vascular diseases.
3. The response of CVP to fluid is variable and must be measured between aliquots.
4. Transfer to intensive care for insertion of a pulmonary artery catheter if volume status remains in doubt.
5. Avoid an excessively high CVP which may signify RV dysfunction due to overdistension.

Which fluid?

1. Packed red blood cells have a high haematocrit. Additional fluid may be required for a volume response.
2. Crystalloid fluids (e.g. 0.9% saline, 5% glucose) are not an efficient means of expanding the plasma volume. Approximately 3/4 of a crystalloid infusion is quickly lost from the plasma.
3. Gelatin solutions (e.g. Gelofusine) can be recommended for short term plasma expansion in simple hypovolaemia and hydroxyethyl starch solution (e.g. Elohes) when there is capillary leak.

Bibliography

Haupt MT, Rackow EC. Colloid osmotic pressure and fluid resuscitation with hetastarch, albumin, and saline solutions. *Crit Care Med* 1982; **10**:159

Imm A, Carlson RW. Fluid resuscitation in circulatory shock. *Crit Care Clin* 1993; **9**:313

Lazrove S, Waxman K, Shippy C, Shoemaker WC. Hemodynamic, blood volume and oxygen transport responses to albumin and hydroxyethyl starch infusions in critically ill postoperative patients. *Crit Care Med* 1980; **8**:302

Lundsgaard Hansen P, Pappova E. Colloids versus crystalloids as volume substitutes: clinical relevance of the serum oncotic pressure. *Ann Clin Res* 1981; **133**:5

Manny J, Grindlinger GA, Dennis RC, *et al.* Myocardial performance curves as a guide to volume therapy. *Surg Gynecol Obstet* 1979; **149**:863

Sturm JA, Wisner DH. Fluid resuscitation of hypovolemia. *Intensive Care Med* 1985; **11**:227

Webb AR, Barclay SA, Bennett ED. In vitro colloid osmotic pressure of commonly used plasma substitutes: a study of the diffusibility of colloid molecules. *Intensive Care Med* 1989; **15**:116

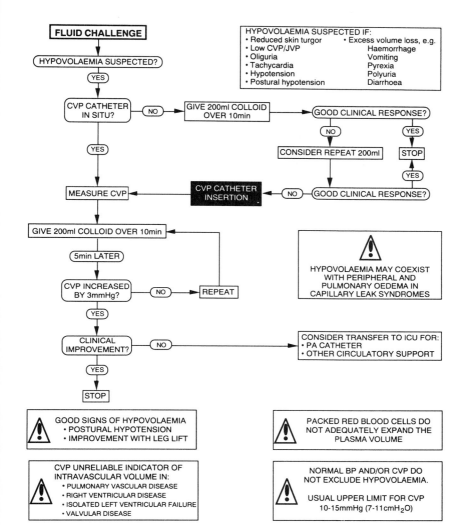

FLUID CHALLENGE

HYPOVOLAEMIA SUSPECTED?
→ YES

HYPOVOLAEMIA SUSPECTED IF:
- Reduced skin turgor
- Low CVP/JVP
- Oliguria
- Tachycardia
- Hypotension
- Postural hypotension
- Excess volume loss, e.g.
  Haemorrhage
  Vomiting
  Pyrexia
  Polyuria
  Diarrhoea

CVP CATHETER IN SITU? — NO → GIVE 200ml COLLOID OVER 10min → GOOD CLINICAL RESPONSE?

GOOD CLINICAL RESPONSE? — NO → CONSIDER REPEAT 200ml
GOOD CLINICAL RESPONSE? — YES → STOP

CONSIDER REPEAT 200ml → GOOD CLINICAL RESPONSE? — YES → STOP

CVP CATHETER INSERTION — NO → GOOD CLINICAL RESPONSE?

CVP CATHETER IN SITU? → YES → MEASURE CVP ← CVP CATHETER INSERTION

MEASURE CVP → GIVE 200ml COLLOID OVER 10min

5min LATER

CVP INCREASED BY 3mmHg? — NO → REPEAT
→ YES

CLINICAL IMPROVEMENT? — NO → CONSIDER TRANSFER TO ICU FOR:
- PA CATHETER
- OTHER CIRCULATORY SUPPORT
→ YES

STOP

⚠ HYPOVOLAEMIA MAY COEXIST WITH PERIPHERAL AND PULMONARY OEDEMA IN CAPILLARY LEAK SYNDROMES

⚠ GOOD SIGNS OF HYPOVOLAEMIA
- POSTURAL HYPOTENSION
- IMPROVEMENT WITH LEG LIFT

⚠ PACKED RED BLOOD CELLS DO NOT ADEQUATELY EXPAND THE PLASMA VOLUME

⚠ CVP UNRELIABLE INDICATOR OF INTRAVASCULAR VOLUME IN:
- PULMONARY VASCULAR DISEASE
- RIGHT VENTRICULAR DISEASE
- ISOLATED LEFT VENTRICULAR FAILURE
- VALVULAR DISEASE

⚠ NORMAL BP AND/OR CVP DO NOT EXCLUDE HYPOVOLAEMIA.

USUAL UPPER LIMIT FOR CVP
10-15mmHg (7-11cmH$_2$O)

2. Respiratory

2.1 Upper airway obstruction

Causes
1. Care should be exercised when moving the neck if a history of trauma is given.
2. Initially, patients may only be symptomatic during exertion.
3. Inspiratory stridor is an ominous sign.
4. Epiglottitis can also occur in adults.

Reversible obstruction
1. Head and neck positioning is important in a comatose patient to prevent obstructed breathing by the tongue/epiglottis.
2. Snoring is an indication of partial obstruction.
3. An oropharyngeal (Guedel) or nasopharyngeal airway may assist in keeping the airway patent.

Management
1. All patients with respiratory obstruction (even mild cases) should be admitted and monitored in a High Dependency Unit/ICU environment as rapid deterioration may occur.
2. The anaesthetist ± ENT surgeon should be contacted at an early stage. It is safer to intubate/perform a tracheostomy as an elective procedure.
3. Heliox (50% helium:50% oxygen) reduces the air viscosity and eases breathing. It is often available in Casualty or Obstetric departments.
4. The Heimlich manoeuvre consists of a short, sharp epigastric thrust to generate an increase in intrathoracic pressure and a forced expiration with, hopefully, ejection of the foreign body from the major airways. (An alternative technique in smaller, lighter patients (usually children) is to hold them upside down and thump the posterior chest in an attempt to dislodge the foreign body.)

Bibliography
Andreassen UK, Baer S, Nielsen TG, *et al.* Acute epiglottitis — 25 years' experience with nasotracheal intubation, current management policy and future trends. *J Laryngol Otol* 1992; **106**:1072
Denholm S, Rivron RP. Acute epiglottitis in adults: a potentially lethal cause of sore throat. *J R Coll Surg Edinb* 1992; **37**:333
Lerner DM, Deeb Z. Acute upper airway obstruction resulting from systemic diseases. *South Med J* 1993; **86**: 623

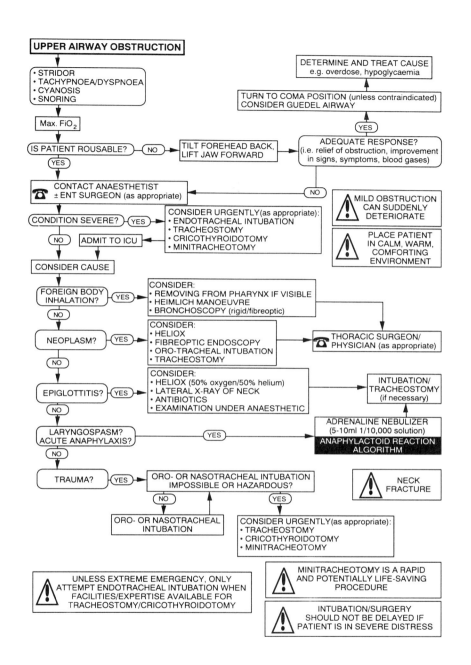

UPPER AIRWAY OBSTRUCTION

- STRIDOR
- TACHYPNOEA/DYSPNOEA
- CYANOSIS
- SNORING

Max. FiO$_2$

IS PATIENT ROUSABLE? — NO → TILT FOREHEAD BACK, LIFT JAW FORWARD

YES

☎ CONTACT ANAESTHETIST ± ENT SURGEON (as appropriate)

CONDITION SEVERE? — YES → CONSIDER URGENTLY (as appropriate):
- ENDOTRACHEAL INTUBATION
- TRACHEOSTOMY
- CRICOTHYROIDOTOMY
- MINITRACHEOTOMY

NO → ADMIT TO ICU

CONSIDER CAUSE

FOREIGN BODY INHALATION? — YES → CONSIDER:
- REMOVING FROM PHARYNX IF VISIBLE
- HEIMLICH MANOEUVRE
- BRONCHOSCOPY (rigid/fibreoptic)

NO

NEOPLASM? — YES → CONSIDER:
- HELIOX
- FIBREOPTIC ENDOSCOPY
- ORO-TRACHEAL INTUBATION
- TRACHEOSTOMY

NO

EPIGLOTTITIS? — YES → CONSIDER:
- HELIOX (50% oxygen/50% helium)
- LATERAL X-RAY OF NECK
- ANTIBIOTICS
- EXAMINATION UNDER ANAESTHETIC

NO

LARYNGOSPASM? ACUTE ANAPHYLAXIS? — YES →

NO

TRAUMA? — YES → ORO- OR NASOTRACHEAL INTUBATION IMPOSSIBLE OR HAZARDOUS?

NO → ORO- OR NASOTRACHEAL INTUBATION

YES → CONSIDER URGENTLY (as appropriate):
- TRACHEOSTOMY
- CRICOTHYROIDOTOMY
- MINITRACHEOTOMY

DETERMINE AND TREAT CAUSE
e.g. overdose, hypoglycaemia

TURN TO COMA POSITION (unless contraindicated) CONSIDER GUEDEL AIRWAY

YES

ADEQUATE RESPONSE? (i.e. relief of obstruction, improvement in signs, symptoms, blood gases)

NO

⚠ MILD OBSTRUCTION CAN SUDDENLY DETERIORATE

⚠ PLACE PATIENT IN CALM, WARM, COMFORTING ENVIRONMENT

☎ THORACIC SURGEON/ PHYSICIAN (as appropriate)

INTUBATION/ TRACHEOSTOMY (if necessary)

ADRENALINE NEBULIZER (5-10ml 1/10,000 solution)

ANAPHYLACTOID REACTION ALGORITHM

⚠ NECK FRACTURE

⚠ UNLESS EXTREME EMERGENCY, ONLY ATTEMPT ENDOTRACHEAL INTUBATION WHEN FACILITIES/EXPERTISE AVAILABLE FOR TRACHEOSTOMY/CRICOTHYROIDOTOMY

⚠ MINITRACHEOTOMY IS A RAPID AND POTENTIALLY LIFE-SAVING PROCEDURE

⚠ INTUBATION/SURGERY SHOULD NOT BE DELAYED IF PATIENT IS IN SEVERE DISTRESS

9

2.2 Acute dyspnoea

1. The priority is to resuscitate the patient promptly and adequately.

Oxygen therapy

1. Give high concentration, high flow oxygen by 60% Ventimask, or by tight fitting mask and reservoir bag. Do not use standard (Hudson) masks as these give unreliable oxygen concentrations.
2. All patients should receive high concentration, high flow oxygen except the small proportion with Type II (chronic hypoxaemic, hypercapnic) respiratory failure [see algorithm 2.5].
3. In the less dyspnoeic patient a lower FiO_2 (0.28–0.4%) can be given provided repeated blood gas analysis/pulse oximetry confirms normoxaemia.

Causes

1. Dyspnoea may be due to dual pathologies causing a mixed respiratory and metabolic acidosis e.g. dehydration and chest infection. Arterial blood gas analysis will reveal this.
2. Psychiatric causes of hyperventilation are only made after excluding organic causes.

Bibliography
Ogilvie C. Dyspnoea. *BMJ* 1983; **287**:160

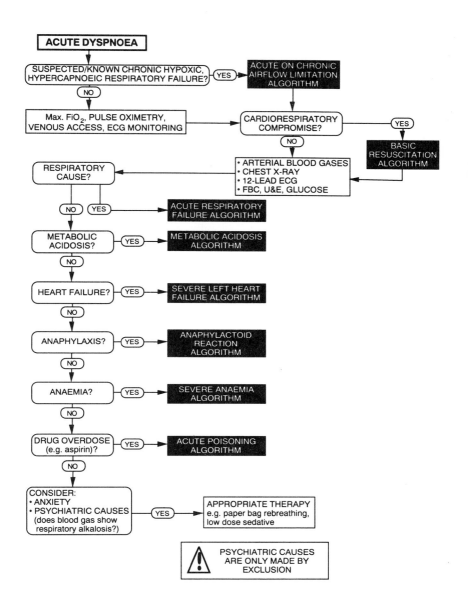

ACUTE DYSPNOEA

SUSPECTED/KNOWN CHRONIC HYPOXIC, HYPERCAPNOEIC RESPIRATORY FAILURE? — YES → ACUTE ON CHRONIC AIRFLOW LIMITATION ALGORITHM

NO

Max. FiO$_2$, PULSE OXIMETRY, VENOUS ACCESS, ECG MONITORING → CARDIORESPIRATORY COMPROMISE? — YES

NO

BASIC RESUSCITATION ALGORITHM

• ARTERIAL BLOOD GASES
• CHEST X-RAY
• 12-LEAD ECG
• FBC, U&E, GLUCOSE

RESPIRATORY CAUSE?

NO   YES → ACUTE RESPIRATORY FAILURE ALGORITHM

METABOLIC ACIDOSIS? — YES → METABOLIC ACIDOSIS ALGORITHM

NO

HEART FAILURE? — YES → SEVERE LEFT HEART FAILURE ALGORITHM

NO

ANAPHYLAXIS? — YES → ANAPHYLACTOID REACTION ALGORITHM

NO

ANAEMIA? — YES → SEVERE ANAEMIA ALGORITHM

NO

DRUG OVERDOSE (e.g. aspirin)? — YES → ACUTE POISONING ALGORITHM

NO

CONSIDER:
• ANXIETY
• PSYCHIATRIC CAUSES (does blood gas show respiratory alkalosis?) — YES → APPROPRIATE THERAPY e.g. paper bag rebreathing, low dose sedative

⚠ PSYCHIATRIC CAUSES ARE ONLY MADE BY EXCLUSION

11

2.3 Acute Respiratory Failure

1. The priority is to resuscitate the patient promptly and adequately.
2. Respiratory failure may be manifest as either a low PaO_2 and/or a high $PaCO_2$.
3. A normal reading on pulse oximetry does not exclude respiratory failure as hypercapnia may often precede hypoxaemia. At least one arterial blood gas sample is mandatory.

Adult respiratory distress syndrome (ARDS)

1. ARDS is the pulmonary manifestation of multiple organ failure.
2. It is characterized by hypoxaemia, bilateral pulmonary infiltrates on chest X-ray, and non-elevated pulmonary artery wedge pressures (thus excluding cardiogenic causes of pulmonary oedema) following hours to days after a severe insult e.g. infection, trauma, pancreatitis.
3. It occurs as a consequence of activation of endogenous inflammatory pathways.
4. Histology reveals endothelial disruption, fibrosis, white cell and platelet aggregation, and interstitial oedema.
5. Treatment consists of removing the cause where possible (antibiotics, drainage of pus, debridement of necrotic tissue, fixation of fractures) and supportive care (usually mechanical ventilation) until recovery occurs. At present no specific treatment exists.
6. Fluid and inotrope management remains controversial. It is generally accepted that tissue oxygen delivery should be sufficient to maintain adequate organ perfusion though when severe hypoxaemia is present a degree of hypovolaemia may be necessary.

Continuous positive airways pressure (CPAP)

1. CPAP is provided by a circuit carrying a high flow air–oxygen mix to the patient who exhales against a valve thereby preventing intrathoracic pressure returning to atmospheric pressure at the end of expiration.
2. The positive pressure is continually exerted, keeping alveoli open during expiration and preventing microatelectasis. This improves oxygenation, reduces the work of breathing and lowers right ventricular preload. Therefore it is also beneficial in heart failure.
3. As CPAP increases the functional residual capacity (FRC) it should only be used by experienced clinicians in patients with an increased FRC e.g. patients with asthma, emphysema . . .
4. The gas flow rate should exceed the peak inspiratory flow rate of the patient to prevent closure of the CPAP valve during inspiration.

Bibliography

Benhamou D, Girault C, Faure C, *et al.* Nasal mask ventilation in acute respiratory failure. *Chest* 1992; **102**: 912

Elliot MW, Steven MH, Phillips GD, Branthwaite MA. Non-invasive mechanical ventilation for acute respiratory failure. *BMJ* 1990; **300**: 358

Hollingsworth HM, Irwin RS. Acute respiratory failure in pregnancy. *Clin Chest Med* 1992; **13**: 723

Kelly BJ, Luce JM. The diagnosis and management of neuromuscular diseases causing respiratory failure. *Chest* 1991; **99**: 1485

Macnaughton PD, Evans TW. Management of adult respiratory distress syndrome. *Lancet* 1992; **339**: 469

Wedzicha W. Nasal ventilation, *Br J Hosp Med* 1992; **47**: 257

Wysocki M, Tric L, Wolff MA, Gertner J, Millet H, Herman B. Noninvasive pressure support ventilation in patients with acute respiratory failure. *Chest* 1993; **103**: 907

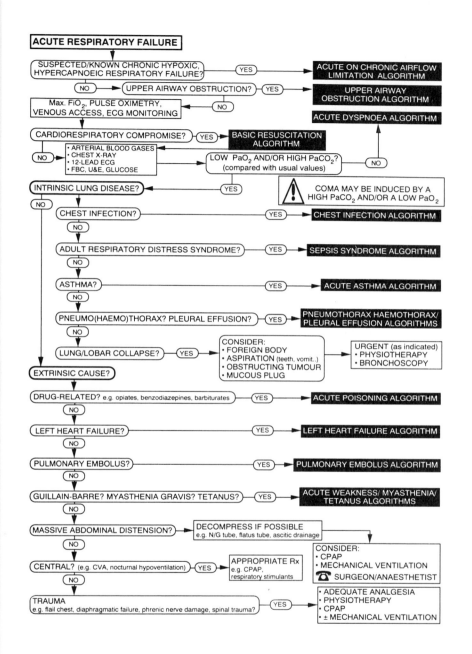

ACUTE RESPIRATORY FAILURE

SUSPECTED/KNOWN CHRONIC HYPOXIC, HYPERCAPNOEIC RESPIRATORY FAILURE? — YES → **ACUTE ON CHRONIC AIRFLOW LIMITATION ALGORITHM**

NO → UPPER AIRWAY OBSTRUCTION? — YES → **UPPER AIRWAY OBSTRUCTION ALGORITHM**

Max. FiO$_2$, PULSE OXIMETRY, VENOUS ACCESS, ECG MONITORING — NO

ACUTE DYSPNOEA ALGORITHM

CARDIORESPIRATORY COMPROMISE? — YES → **BASIC RESUSCITATION ALGORITHM**

NO →
- ARTERIAL BLOOD GASES
- CHEST X-RAY
- 12-LEAD ECG
- FBC, U&E, GLUCOSE

→ LOW PaO$_2$ AND/OR HIGH PaCO$_2$? (compared with usual values) — NO

INTRINSIC LUNG DISEASE? ← YES

⚠ COMA MAY BE INDUCED BY A HIGH PaCO$_2$ AND/OR A LOW PaO$_2$

NO

CHEST INFECTION? — YES → **CHEST INFECTION ALGORITHM**

NO

ADULT RESPIRATORY DISTRESS SYNDROME? — YES → **SEPSIS SYNDROME ALGORITHM**

NO

ASTHMA? — YES → **ACUTE ASTHMA ALGORITHM**

NO

PNEUMO(HAEMO)THORAX? PLEURAL EFFUSION? — YES → **PNEUMOTHORAX HAEMOTHORAX/ PLEURAL EFFUSION ALGORITHMS**

NO

LUNG/LOBAR COLLAPSE? — YES → CONSIDER:
- FOREIGN BODY
- ASPIRATION (teeth, vomit..)
- OBSTRUCTING TUMOUR
- MUCOUS PLUG

→ URGENT (as indicated)
- PHYSIOTHERAPY
- BRONCHOSCOPY

EXTRINSIC CAUSE?

DRUG-RELATED? e.g. opiates, benzodiazepines, barbiturates — YES → **ACUTE POISONING ALGORITHM**

NO

LEFT HEART FAILURE? — YES → **LEFT HEART FAILURE ALGORITHM**

NO

PULMONARY EMBOLUS? — YES → **PULMONARY EMBOLUS ALGORITHM**

NO

GUILLAIN-BARRE? MYASTHENIA GRAVIS? TETANUS? — YES → **ACUTE WEAKNESS/ MYASTHENIA/ TETANUS ALGORITHMS**

NO

MASSIVE ABDOMINAL DISTENSION? → DECOMPRESS IF POSSIBLE e.g. N/G tube, flatus tube, ascitic drainage

NO

CENTRAL? (e.g. CVA, nocturnal hypoventilation) — YES → APPROPRIATE Rx e.g. CPAP, respiratory stimulants

NO

CONSIDER:
- CPAP
- MECHANICAL VENTILATION
- ☎ SURGEON/ANAESTHETIST

TRAUMA e.g. flail chest, diaphragmatic failure, phrenic nerve damage, spinal trauma? — YES →
- ADEQUATE ANALGESIA
- PHYSIOTHERAPY
- CPAP
- ± MECHANICAL VENTILATION

2.4 Acute asthma

Severity
1. Mortality from asthma has increased and is often avoidable by early and aggressive therapy.
2. Two groups of patients with severe acute asthma may be identified:
   - insidious deterioration leading to exhaustion
   - acute catastrophic bronchospasm with early asphyxiation
3. Patients with marked 'morning dipping' are at risk of sudden acute catastrophic attacks.
4. A peak expiratory flow rate (PEFR) below 80 litres/min and a previous history of severe asthma requiring mechanical ventilation are indicators that the patient may require mechanical ventilation.
5. Consider pneumothorax if rapid deterioration occurs.

Therapy
1. A high $PaCO_2$ in acute asthma is not, in general, a contraindication to high FiO_2 therapy.
2. Treatment is required for both bronchospasm and inflammation.
3. Patients who develop respiratory muscle fatigue may avoid mechanical ventilation with the cautious use of CPAP to reduce the work of breathing. However, CPAP should only be used in asthmatics by clinicians experienced in its use.
4. Careful attention to hydration and humidification is required to avoid mucus plugging.
5. Intubation and mechanical ventilation of the acute asthmatic is a potentially hazardous procedure. An experienced anaesthetist should be called (if time allows).
6. Unless responding to a β-agonist nebulizer ± 40 mg prednisolone (i.e. becoming virtually asymptomatic with a PEFR ≥ 75% of normal) and able to be supervised at home, the patient must be admitted, at least for overnight observation and treatment (see morning dipping above).
7. Ipratropium nebulizers, if used, should be given with $β_2$ agonist nebulizers.

Monitoring
1. The patient should always be observed in a warm, quiet, well-monitored area.
2. A fall in PaO_2 is generally seen at a late stage. Increasing fatigue and mental obtundation, and a normal/high $PaCO_2$ are indicators of increasing severity. Such patients should be transferred to the ICU.

Bibliography
Benatar S. Fatal asthma. *N Engl J Med* 1986; **314**:423
Branthwaite MA. The intensive care of asthma. *Brit J Hosp Med* 1985; **34**:331
British Thoracic Society & others. Guidelines for the management of asthma: a summary. *BMJ* 1993; **306**: 776
Burney PGJ. Asthma mortality in England and Wales: evidence for a further increase, 1979–84. *Lancet* 1986; **ii**:323
Freedman AR, Lavietes MH. Energy requirements of the respiratory musculature in asthma. *Am J Med* 1986; **80**:215
Gluck GH, Onorato DJ, Cantriotta J. Helium–oxygen mixtures in intubated patients with status asthmaticus and respiratory acidosis. *Chest* 1990; **98**: 693
Henderson A, Wright M. Status asthmaticus: experience of 100 consecutive admissions to an intensive care unit. *Clinical Intensive Care* 1992; **3**: 148
Jones D. Can we recognise very severe asthma? *Thorax* 1978; **33**:675
Pearson MG, Spence DPS, Ryland I, Harrison BDW. Value of pulsus paradoxus in assessing acute severe asthma. *BMJ* 1993; **307**: 659

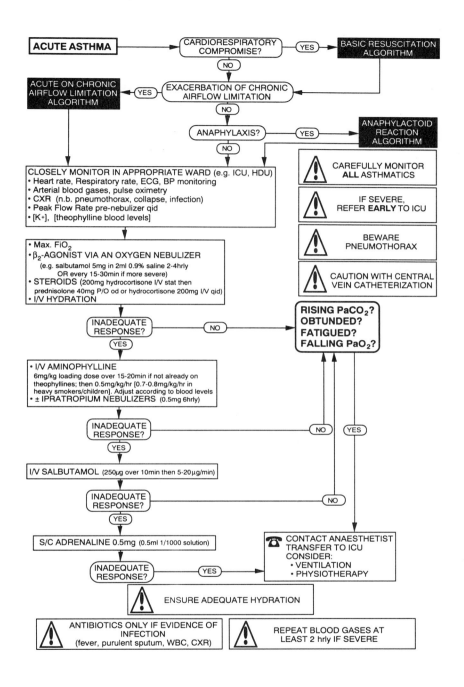

ACUTE ASTHMA

CARDIORESPIRATORY COMPROMISE? — YES → BASIC RESUSCITATION ALGORITHM

NO

ACUTE ON CHRONIC AIRFLOW LIMITATION ALGORITHM ← YES — EXACERBATION OF CHRONIC AIRFLOW LIMITATION

NO

ANAPHYLAXIS? — YES → ANAPHYLACTOID REACTION ALGORITHM

NO

⚠ CAREFULLY MONITOR **ALL** ASTHMATICS

⚠ IF SEVERE, REFER **EARLY** TO ICU

⚠ BEWARE PNEUMOTHORAX

⚠ CAUTION WITH CENTRAL VEIN CATHETERIZATION

CLOSELY MONITOR IN APPROPRIATE WARD (e.g. ICU, HDU)
• Heart rate, Respiratory rate, ECG, BP monitoring
• Arterial blood gases, pulse oximetry
• CXR (n.b. pneumothorax, collapse, infection)
• Peak Flow Rate pre-nebulizer qid
• [K+], [theophylline blood levels]

• Max. FiO_2
• β_2-AGONIST VIA AN OXYGEN NEBULIZER
(e.g. salbutamol 5mg in 2ml 0.9% saline 2-4hrly
OR every 15-30min if more severe)
• STEROIDS (200mg hydrocortisone I/V stat then
prednisolone 40mg P/O od or hydrocortisone 200mg I/V qid)
• I/V HYDRATION

INADEQUATE RESPONSE? — NO →

YES

RISING $PaCO_2$?
OBTUNDED?
FATIGUED?
FALLING PaO_2?

• I/V AMINOPHYLLINE
6mg/kg loading dose over 15-20min if not already on
theophyllines; then 0.5mg/kg/hr [0.7-0.8mg/kg/hr in
heavy smokers/children]. Adjust according to blood levels
• ± IPRATROPIUM NEBULIZERS (0.5mg 6hrly)

INADEQUATE RESPONSE? — NO / YES

YES

I/V SALBUTAMOL (250µg over 10min then 5-20µg/min)

INADEQUATE RESPONSE? — NO

YES

S/C ADRENALINE 0.5mg (0.5ml 1/1000 solution)

INADEQUATE RESPONSE? — YES →

☎ CONTACT ANAESTHETIST
TRANSFER TO ICU
CONSIDER:
• VENTILATION
• PHYSIOTHERAPY

⚠ ENSURE ADEQUATE HYDRATION

⚠ ANTIBIOTICS ONLY IF EVIDENCE OF INFECTION
(fever, purulent sputum, WBC, CXR)

⚠ REPEAT BLOOD GASES AT LEAST 2 hrly IF SEVERE

Rea HH, Scragg R, Jackson R, Beaglehole R, Fenwick J, Sutherland DC. A case-control study of deaths from asthma. *Thorax* 1986; **41**:833

Shivaram U, Miro AM, Cash ME, Finch PJ, Heurich AE, Kamholz SL. Cardiorespiratory responses to continuous positive airway pressure in acute asthma. *J Crit Care* 1993; **8**:87

2.5 Acute on chronic airflow limitation

Management
1. Repeated blood gas analysis at regular intervals aids management decisions.
2. Use a Ventimask to ensure known FiO_2. Keep mask in place.
3. Repeat blood gas analysis 10–15 minutes after change in FiO_2.
4. Give nebulizers in air but ensure adequate oxygenation first.
5. An early decision should be made by a senior doctor on the extent of therapy, e.g. mechanical ventilation. If the history is unclear, patients should be mechanically ventilated if necessary.
6. If the patient is moribund and hypoxaemic then high concentration, high flow oxygen should not be withheld while the anaesthetist is being awaited for intubation. Be prepared to use a Manual Resuscitation Bag (e.g. Ambu bag) if patient becomes apnoeic/bradypnoeic in interim.
7. The tiring patient not for mechanical ventilation may respond to a doxapram infusion and/or non-invasive modes of ventilation e.g. BIPAP, CPAP. These modes reduce the work of breathing but should only be used in these patients by clinicians experienced in their use.
8. Baseline levels of PaO_2 and $PaCO_2$ in these patients are abnormal and the patient has usually compensated either fully or partially e.g. by raising plasma bicarbonate, secondary polycythaemia. It is unnecessary to attempt to improve the blood gases beyond chronic baseline levels.

Complications
1. Consider pneumothorax and lung collapse as causes of acute deterioration.
2. Bullae are more common in this patient group and may be mistaken for pneumothorax. Insertion of a chest drain into a bulla may prove fatal.

Bibliography
Benhamou D, Girault C, Faure C, *et al.* Nasal mask ventilation in acute respiratory failure. *Chest* 1992; **102**: 912
Bott J, Carroll MP, Conway JH, *et al.* Randomised controlled trial of nasal ventilation in acute ventilatory failure due to chronic obstructive airways disease. *Lancet* 1993; **341**: 1555
Elliot MW, Steven MH, Phillips GD, Branthwaite MA. Non-invasive mechanical ventilation for acute respiratory failure. *BMJ* 1990; **300**: 358
Esteban A, Cerda E, De La Cal MA, Lorente JA. Hemodynamic effects of oxygen therapy in patients with acute exacerbations of chronic obstructive pulmonary disease. *Chest* 1993; **104**: 471
Jeffrey AA, Warren PM, Flenley DC. Acute hypercapnic respiratory failure in patients with chronic obstructive lung disease: risk factors and use of guidelines for management. *Thorax* 1992; **47**: 34
Meduri GU, Abou-Shala N, Jones CB, Leeper KV, Wunderink RG. Noninvasive face mask mechanical ventilation in patients with acute hypercapnic respiratory failure. *Chest* 1991; **100**: 445
Vitacca M, Rubini F, Foglio K, Scalvini S, Nava S, Ambrosino N. Non-invasive modalities of positive pressure ventilation improve the outcome of acute exacerbations in COLD patients. *Intensive Care Med* 1992; **19**: 450

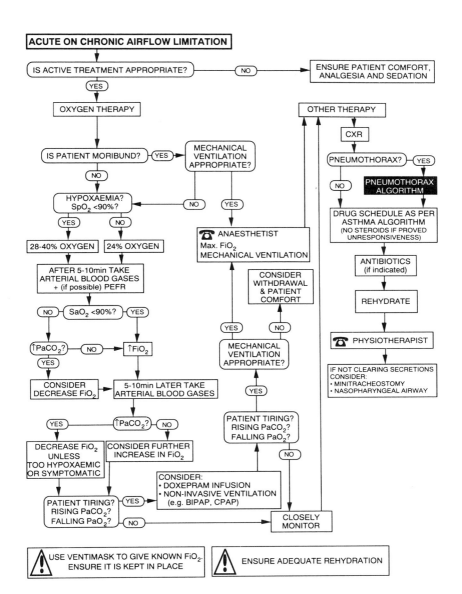

ACUTE ON CHRONIC AIRFLOW LIMITATION

IS ACTIVE TREATMENT APPROPRIATE? —NO→ ENSURE PATIENT COMFORT, ANALGESIA AND SEDATION

YES

OXYGEN THERAPY

IS PATIENT MORIBUND? —YES→ MECHANICAL VENTILATION APPROPRIATE?

NO

HYPOXAEMIA? SpO$_2$ <90%? ←NO

YES / NO

28-40% OXYGEN | 24% OXYGEN

AFTER 5-10min TAKE ARTERIAL BLOOD GASES + (if possible) PEFR

NO— SaO$_2$ <90%? —YES

↑PaCO$_2$? —NO→ ↑FiO$_2$

YES

CONSIDER DECREASE FiO$_2$ | 5-10min LATER TAKE ARTERIAL BLOOD GASES

YES— ↑PaCO$_2$? —NO

DECREASE FiO$_2$ UNLESS TOO HYPOXAEMIC OR SYMPTOMATIC | CONSIDER FURTHER INCREASE IN FiO$_2$

PATIENT TIRING? RISING PaCO$_2$? FALLING PaO$_2$? —YES→ CONSIDER:
• DOXEPRAM INFUSION
• NON-INVASIVE VENTILATION (e.g. BIPAP, CPAP)

NO→ CLOSELY MONITOR

MECHANICAL VENTILATION APPROPRIATE? — NO / YES

☎ ANAESTHETIST Max. FiO$_2$ MECHANICAL VENTILATION

CONSIDER WITHDRAWAL & PATIENT COMFORT

YES / NO

MECHANICAL VENTILATION APPROPRIATE?

YES

PATIENT TIRING? RISING PaCO$_2$? FALLING PaO$_2$? —NO

OTHER THERAPY

CXR

PNEUMOTHORAX? —YES→ PNEUMOTHORAX ALGORITHM

NO

DRUG SCHEDULE AS PER ASTHMA ALGORITHM (NO STEROIDS IF PROVED UNRESPONSIVENESS)

ANTIBIOTICS (if indicated)

REHYDRATE

☎ PHYSIOTHERAPIST

IF NOT CLEARING SECRETIONS CONSIDER:
• MINITRACHEOSTOMY
• NASOPHARYNGEAL AIRWAY

⚠ USE VENTIMASK TO GIVE KNOWN FiO$_2$. ENSURE IT IS KEPT IN PLACE

⚠ ENSURE ADEQUATE REHYDRATION

17

2.6 Acute chest infection

General management of chest infection

1. In previously healthy patients oxygen therapy should be started in high concentration (FiO_2 at least 0.4–0.6).
2. If SpO_2 >90% cannot be achieved in a previously healthy patient, $PaCO_2$ rises or patient fatigues, transfer to intensive care and consider early ventilation or CPAP.
3. Cough should not be suppressed if sputum is present.
4. Hypovolaemia is commonly associated with chest infection; failure to correct may be associated with:
   - circulatory collapse
   - retention of tenacious sputum
   - multiple organ failure

Acute bronchitis

1. In previously healthy patients acute bronchitis is usually viral requiring symptomatic treatment only.
2. In patients with chronic lung disease acute bronchitis may be viral or bacterial. Viral infection is often confused by the presence of *H. influenzae* or *Strep. pneumoniae* in sputum.
3. Secondary bacterial infection is common in patients with acute bronchitis and chronic lung disease.

Acute pneumonia

1. Bacteriological diagnosis on sputum and blood cultures should ideally be made before starting antibiotic therapy. However, most patients requiring hospital admission require antibiotic therapy immediately.
2. Bacteriological diagnosis is often difficult to make if patients have been treated with antibiotics prior to hospital presentation.
3. If patients are severely ill on clinical presentation or there is underlying chronic lung disease, intravenous antibiotic therapy should be started empirically (choices as in algorithm).
4. Lobar pneumonia is commonly due to *Strep. pneumoniae* but *Klebsiella pneumoniae* is a rare cause of community-acquired lobar pneumonia requiring prolonged antibiotic therapy with ceftazidime and gentamicin.
5. Antibiotic therapy to cover *Staph. aureus* should be considered in patients with pneumonia complicating influenza.
6. Failure to respond to initial antibiotic therapy should signal consideration of TB.
7. Diagnosis of atypical pneumonia should be based upon:
   - known community outbreaks
   - high degree of suspicion
   - rise in specific antibody titres (often retrospective)
   - urinary antigen test in Legionella pneumonia
8. In the immunosuppressed patient bronchoscopic isolation of organisms may be required:
   - fungal isolates treated with amphotericin B and fluconazole
   - *Pneumocystis carinii* treated with high dose cotrimoxazole (120 mg/day I/V) and high dose methylprednisolone (1 g/day I/V for 3 days)

Viral pneumonia

1. Viral pneumonia is diagnosed by exclusion. It is not confirmed by the absence of bacterial isolates.
2. Clinical features vary but may include a prodromal upper respiratory tract infection, acute exanthemata and lymphocytosis.
3. In the immunocompromised viral pneumonia due to varicella or *Herpes simplex* should be treated with acyclovir (10 mg/kg tid I/V)
4. In the immunocompromised ganciclovir should be considered for severe cytomegalovirus (CMV) pneumonia.

Initial antibiotic dosages	
Ampicillin	500 mg–1 g I/V 6 hrly
Benzylpenicillin	1.2 g I/V 6 hrly (2 hrly for pneumococcal pneumonia)
Cefuroxime	1.5 g I/V 8 hrly (750 mg I/V 8 hrly if less severe)
Ceftazidime	2 g I/V 8 hrly
Clindamycin	300–600 mg I/V 6 hrly
Erythromycin	1 g I/V 6-12 hrly (500 mg P/O 6 hrly if less severe)
Flucloxacillin	2 g I/V 6 hrly (500 mg–1 g P/O 6 hrly if less severe)
Gentamicin	1.5 mg/kg stat. (thereafter by levels—usually 80 mg 8 hrly)
Metronidazole	500 mg I/V 8 hrly or 1 g P/R 12 hrly

1. These dosages may need adjusting in the presence of renal or hepatic failure.

Bibliography

British Thoracic Society. Guidelines for the management of community-acquired pneumonia in adults admitted to hospital. *Br J Hosp Med* 1993; **49**:346

British Thoracic Society Research Committee and the Public Health Laboratory Service. The aetiology, management and outcome of severe community-acquired pneumonia on the intensive care unit. *Respir Med* 1992; **86**: 7

Meyer RD. Legionella infections: a review of five years of research. *Rev Infect Dis* 1983; **5**:258

Park GR, Drummond GB, Lamb D, *et al.* Disseminated aspergillosis in patients with respiratory, renal and hepatic failure. *Lancet* 1982; **ii**:179

Wilson APR. Antibiotic therapy in the critically ill. In: Tinker J and Zapol WM (Eds) Care of the critically ill. Springer Verlag, Berlin, 1992, p1145

Winston DJ, Lau WK, Gale RP, Young LS. Trimethoprim/sulfamethoxazole for the treatment of Pneumocystis carinii pneumonia. *Ann Intern Med* 1980; **92**:762

RESPIRATORY

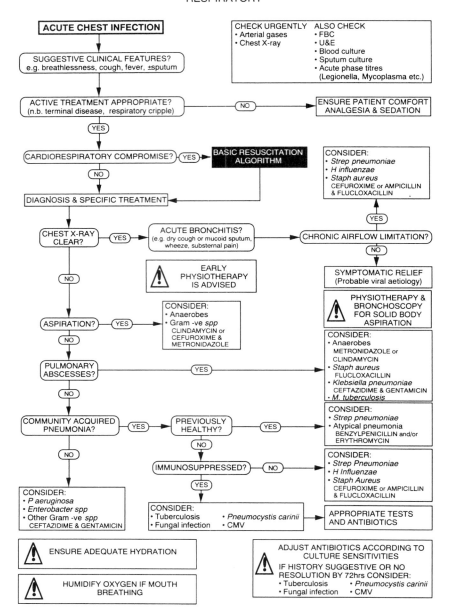

ACUTE CHEST INFECTION

CHECK URGENTLY	ALSO CHECK
• Arterial gases	• FBC
• Chest X-ray	• U&E
	• Blood culture
	• Sputum culture
	• Acute phase titres
	(Legionella, Mycoplasma etc.)

SUGGESTIVE CLINICAL FEATURES?
e.g. breathlessness, cough, fever, ±sputum

ACTIVE TREATMENT APPROPRIATE?
(n.b. terminal disease, respiratory cripple) — NO → ENSURE PATIENT COMFORT ANALGESIA & SEDATION

YES

CARDIORESPIRATORY COMPROMISE? — YES → BASIC RESUSCITATION ALGORITHM

NO

CONSIDER:
• *Strep pneumoniae*
• *H influenzae*
• *Staph aureus*
 CEFUROXIME or AMPICILLIN
 & FLUCLOXACILLIN

DIAGNOSIS & SPECIFIC TREATMENT

CHEST X-RAY CLEAR? — YES → ACUTE BRONCHITIS?
(e.g. dry cough or mucoid sputum, wheeze, substernal pain) → CHRONIC AIRFLOW LIMITATION?

YES

NO

⚠ EARLY PHYSIOTHERAPY IS ADVISED

SYMPTOMATIC RELIEF
(Probable viral aetiology)

⚠ PHYSIOTHERAPY & BRONCHOSCOPY FOR SOLID BODY ASPIRATION

ASPIRATION? — YES → CONSIDER:
• Anaerobes
• Gram -ve *spp*
 CLINDAMYCIN or
 CEFUROXIME &
 METRONIDAZOLE

NO

CONSIDER:
• Anaerobes
 METRONIDAZOLE or
 CLINDAMYCIN
• *Staph aureus*
 FLUCLOXACILLIN
• *Klebsiella pneumoniae*
 CEFTAZIDIME & GENTAMICIN
• *M. tuberculosis*

PULMONARY ABSCESSES? — YES →

NO

COMMUNITY ACQUIRED PNEUMONIA? — YES → PREVIOUSLY HEALTHY? — YES → CONSIDER:
• *Strep pneumoniae*
• Atypical pneumonia
 BENZYLPENICILLIN and/or
 ERYTHROMYCIN

NO

NO

CONSIDER:
• *Strep Pneumoniae*
• *H Influenzae*
• *Staph Aureus*
 CEFUROXIME or AMPICILLIN
 & FLUCLOXACILLIN

IMMUNOSUPPRESSED? — NO →

YES

CONSIDER:
• *P aeruginosa*
• *Enterobacter spp*
• Other Gram -ve *spp*
 CEFTAZIDIME & GENTAMICIN

CONSIDER:
• Tuberculosis   • *Pneumocystis carinii*
• Fungal infection   • CMV

APPROPRIATE TESTS AND ANTIBIOTICS

⚠ ENSURE ADEQUATE HYDRATION

⚠ HUMIDIFY OXYGEN IF MOUTH BREATHING

⚠ ADJUST ANTIBIOTICS ACCORDING TO CULTURE SENSITIVITIES
IF HISTORY SUGGESTIVE OR NO RESOLUTION BY 72hrs CONSIDER:
• Tuberculosis   • *Pneumocystis carinii*
• Fungal infection   • CMV

Notes

2.7/2.8 Pneumothorax/haemothorax/large pleural effusion

Management of pneumothorax

1. The differential diagnosis includes bullous emphysema, pneumatocoele and intrapulmonary cyst. It is important to recognize these conditions and avoid a chest drain unless there is an assured pneumothorax.
2. A pneumothorax may be missed on a supine chest X-ray since the lung edge or an absence of lung markings may not be seen. A hyperlucent lung field, loss of clarity of diaphragm outline, the 'deep sulcus' sign or a particularly clear cardiac margin are suggestive.
3. It may take the lung several weeks to re-expand with a conservatively treated pneumothorax.
4. The lung rarely re-expands on its own if a pneumothorax is associated with underlying diffuse lung disease.
5. All pneumothoraces should be drained in mechanically ventilated patients.
6. All pneumothoraces should be drained prior to any inter-hospital transfer.
7. A pneumothorax which is not causing distress in a young patient could be aspirated rather than drained.

Insertion of a chest drain

1. A chest drain of size 28 French or larger is required for a haemothorax whereas 20 French will suffice for a pure pneumothorax.
2. Insert via the Vth intercostal space in the mid axillary line.
3. Anaesthetize skin and pleura with 1% plain lignocaine. Ensure that air or fluid is aspirated.
4. Make a 1–1.5 cm skin crease incision and create a track with artery forceps and gloved finger to separate muscle fibres and to open pleura.
5. To avoid lung damage insert the drain with the trochar slightly withdrawn. Angle and insert the drain to a correct position. Connect drain to an underwater seal.
6. The chest drain should be directed towards the apex of the lung for a pneumothorax and towards the base of the lung for a haemothorax/pleural effusion.
7. The drain should be well secured to the chest wall by properly placed sutures.
8. After drain insertion always do a chest X-ray to ensure correct placement and lung reinflation.

Management of the chest drain

1. Chest drains do not need to be clamped prior to removal or transport of the patient.
2. Chest drains may be removed in spontaneously breathing patients when the lung has re-expanded and there is no air leak.
3. The risk of lung entrapment and infarction is increased by the practice of chest drain milking and this should be avoided in pneumothorax.
4. Remove chest drains at end-expiration.

Complications of chest drainage

1. Morbidity associated with chest drainage may be up to 10%:
   - damage to intrathoracic viscera or intercostal vessels
   - septic complications
   - chest wall discomfort
   - impaired coughing
   - dislodgement of tube

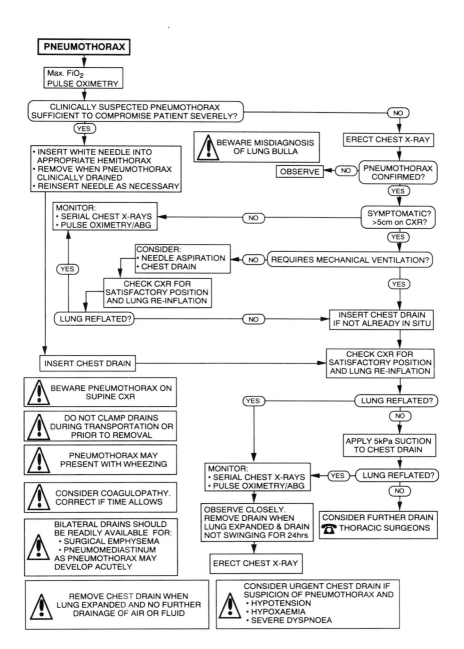

PNEUMOTHORAX

Max. FiO₂
PULSE OXIMETRY

CLINICALLY SUSPECTED PNEUMOTHORAX
SUFFICIENT TO COMPROMISE PATIENT SEVERELY? — NO

YES

ERECT CHEST X-RAY

BEWARE MISDIAGNOSIS
OF LUNG BULLA

- INSERT WHITE NEEDLE INTO
  APPROPRIATE HEMITHORAX
- REMOVE WHEN PNEUMOTHORAX
  CLINICALLY DRAINED
- REINSERT NEEDLE AS NECESSARY

OBSERVE — NO — PNEUMOTHORAX
CONFIRMED?

YES

MONITOR:
- SERIAL CHEST X-RAYS
- PULSE OXIMETRY/ABG — NO — SYMPTOMATIC?
>5cm on CXR?

YES

CONSIDER:
- NEEDLE ASPIRATION
- CHEST DRAIN — NO — REQUIRES MECHANICAL VENTILATION?

YES

YES

CHECK CXR FOR
SATISFACTORY POSITION
AND LUNG RE-INFLATION

LUNG REFLATED? — NO — INSERT CHEST DRAIN
IF NOT ALREADY IN SITU

INSERT CHEST DRAIN — CHECK CXR FOR
SATISFACTORY POSITION
AND LUNG RE-INFLATION

BEWARE PNEUMOTHORAX ON
SUPINE CXR

YES — LUNG REFLATED?

DO NOT CLAMP DRAINS
DURING TRANSPORTATION OR
PRIOR TO REMOVAL

NO

PNEUMOTHORAX MAY
PRESENT WITH WHEEZING

APPLY 5kPa SUCTION
TO CHEST DRAIN

CONSIDER COAGULOPATHY.
CORRECT IF TIME ALLOWS

MONITOR:
- SERIAL CHEST X-RAYS
- PULSE OXIMETRY/ABG — YES — LUNG REFLATED?

NO

BILATERAL DRAINS SHOULD
BE READILY AVAILABLE FOR:
- SURGICAL EMPHYSEMA
- PNEUMOMEDIASTINUM
AS PNEUMOTHORAX MAY
DEVELOP ACUTELY

OBSERVE CLOSELY.
REMOVE DRAIN WHEN
LUNG EXPANDED & DRAIN
NOT SWINGING FOR 24hrs

CONSIDER FURTHER DRAIN
☎ THORACIC SURGEONS

ERECT CHEST X-RAY

REMOVE CHEST DRAIN WHEN
LUNG EXPANDED AND NO FURTHER
DRAINAGE OF AIR OR FLUID

CONSIDER URGENT CHEST DRAIN IF
SUSPICION OF PNEUMOTHORAX AND
- HYPOTENSION
- HYPOXAEMIA
- SEVERE DYSPNOEA

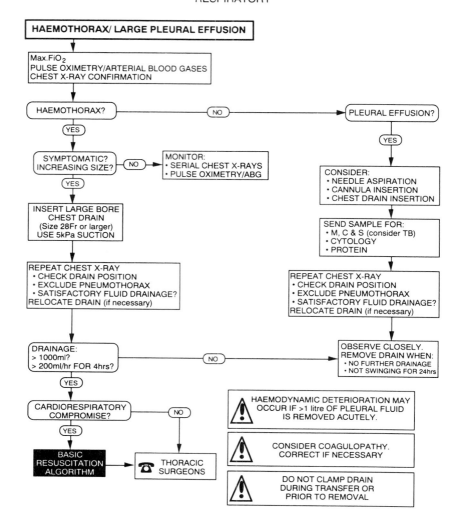

HAEMOTHORAX/ LARGE PLEURAL EFFUSION

Max.FiO$_2$
PULSE OXIMETRY/ARTERIAL BLOOD GASES
CHEST X-RAY CONFIRMATION

HAEMOTHORAX? ──NO──→ PLEURAL EFFUSION?

YES

YES

SYMPTOMATIC? ──NO──→ MONITOR:
INCREASING SIZE? • SERIAL CHEST X-RAYS
• PULSE OXIMETRY/ABG

CONSIDER:
• NEEDLE ASPIRATION
• CANNULA INSERTION
• CHEST DRAIN INSERTION

YES

INSERT LARGE BORE
CHEST DRAIN
(Size 28Fr or larger)
USE 5kPa SUCTION

SEND SAMPLE FOR:
• M, C & S (consider TB)
• CYTOLOGY
• PROTEIN

REPEAT CHEST X-RAY
• CHECK DRAIN POSITION
• EXCLUDE PNEUMOTHORAX
• SATISFACTORY FLUID DRAINAGE?
RELOCATE DRAIN (if necessary)

REPEAT CHEST X-RAY
• CHECK DRAIN POSITION
• EXCLUDE PNEUMOTHORAX
• SATISFACTORY FLUID DRAINAGE?
RELOCATE DRAIN (if necessary)

DRAINAGE:
> 1000ml?
> 200ml/hr FOR 4hrs? ──NO──→ OBSERVE CLOSELY.
REMOVE DRAIN WHEN:
• NO FURTHER DRAINAGE
• NOT SWINGING FOR 24hrs

YES

CARDIORESPIRATORY ──NO──→
COMPROMISE?

YES

BASIC
RESUSCITATION ──→ ☎ THORACIC
ALGORITHM SURGEONS

⚠ HAEMODYNAMIC DETERIORATION MAY
OCCUR IF >1 litre OF PLEURAL FLUID
IS REMOVED ACUTELY.

⚠ CONSIDER COAGULOPATHY.
CORRECT IF NECESSARY

⚠ DO NOT CLAMP DRAIN
DURING TRANSFER OR
PRIOR TO REMOVAL

Bibliography

Cummin A, Smith MJ, Wilson AG. Pneumothorax in the supine patient. *BMJ* 1987; **295**: 591

Gordon R. The deep sulcus sign. *Radiology* 1980; **136**: 25

Gustman P, Yerger L, Wanner A. Immediate cardiovascular effects of tension pneumothorax. *Am Rev Respir Dis* 1983; **127**:171

Minami H, Saka H, Senda K, *et al.* Small caliber catheter drainage for spontaneous pneumothorax. *Am J Med Sci* 1992; **304**: 345

Standards of Care Committee, British Thoracic Society. Guidelines for the management of spontaneous pneumothorax. *BMJ* 1993; **307**: 114 (see also letters: *BMJ;* 1993; **443**)

Tocino IM, Miller MH, Fairfax WR. Distribution of pneumothorax in the supine and semi-recumbent critically ill adult. *AJR* 1985; **144**: 901

Wallis J, Wells F. Chest injuries: diagnosis and management. *Care of the Critically Ill* 1987; **3**: 187

3. Cardiovascular

3.1 Cardiac arrest

Cardiopulmonary resuscitation
1. The effect of cardiac massage is explained by two theories. Cardiac massage at 80–100 compressions/min is a compromise satisfying the cardiac compression and thoracic pump theories. Higher cardiac outputs are generated with higher rates if cardiac compression predominates and with longer compressions if thoracic pumping predominates.
2. Maintenance of good oxygenation by manual ventilation is more important than early intubation.
3. When intubation is attempted it should be effected quickly to avoid hypoxaemia and interruption of CPR.
4. Intramuscular drugs should not be given as perfusion of muscle beds cannot be guaranteed during CPR.
5. Drug therapy for a cardiac arrest should be given via a large vein; vasoconstriction and poor flow create considerable delay in injections given into small peripheral veins reaching the central circulation.
6. There is a delay between defibrillation and return of the ECG trace. CPR should continue during this period.
7. Fixed dilated pupils cannot be used as a prognostic sign during CPR.

Adrenaline
1. The α (vasoconstrictor) effects of adrenaline predominate during resuscitation thus maintaining aortic diastolic blood pressure and coronary and cerebral perfusion.
2. At least $10\,\mu g/kg/5$ min is required for optimal effect in all cardiac arrests, irrespective of rhythm.

Bicarbonate
1. Sodium bicarbonate may exacerbate intracellular and respiratory acidosis.
2. Whereas effective CPR may correct the cause of the metabolic acidosis, sodium bicarbonate does not.
3. Sodium bicarbonate should only be considered if resuscitation is prolonged.
4. If an adequate circulation is difficult to establish, sodium bicarbonate may temporarily correct a potentially lethal pH.

Calcium
1. Reperfusion of ischaemic brain is reduced after calcium has been given.
2. Cytoplasmic calcium accumulation is associated with cell death.
3. Calcium should only be used if there is good evidence of hypocalcaemia (e.g. calcium antagonist drugs) or hyperkalaemia as a cause of the cardiac arrest.

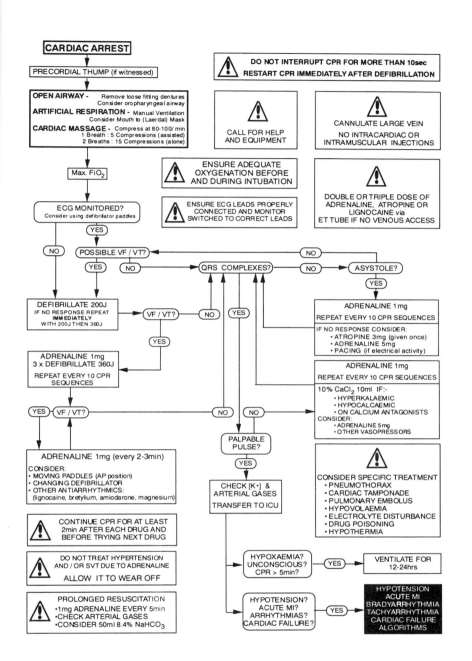

Bibliography

Dembo DH. Calcium in advanced life support. *Crit Care Med* 1981; **9**:358

European Resuscitation Council. Guidelines for advanced cardiac life support. *Resuscitation* 1992; **24**:103

Graf H, Leach W, Arieff Al. Evidence for a detrimental effect of bicarbonate therapy in hypoxic lactic acidosis. *Science* 1985; **227**:754

Halperin HR, Tsitlk JE, Guerci AD, *et al.* Determinants of blood flow to vital organs during cardiopulmonary resuscitation in dogs. *Circulation* 1986; **73**:539

Katz AM, Reuter H. Cellular calcium and cardiac cell death. *Am J Cardiol* 1979; **44**:188

Maier GW, Tyson GS, Olsen CO, *et al.* The physiology of external cardiac massage: High impulse cardiopulmonary resuscitation. *Circulation* 1984; **70**:86

Marsden AK. Basic life support. *BMJ* 1989; **299**:442

Michael JR, Guerci AD, Koehler RC, *et al.* Mechanisms by which epinephrine augments cerebral and myocardial perfusion during cardiopulmonary resuscitation in dogs. *Circulation* 1984; **69**:822

Narins RG, Cohen JJ. Bicarbonate therapy for organic acidosis: The case for its continued use. *Ann Intern Med* 1987; **106**:615

Renekov L. Calcium antagonist drugs—myocardial preservation and reduced vulnerability to ventricular fibrillation during CPR. *Crit Care Med* 1981; **9**:360

Schleien CL, Berkowitz ID, Traystman R, Rogers MC. Controversial issues in cardiopulmonary resuscitation. *Anesthesiology* 1989; **71**:133

Stacpoole PW. Lactic acidosis: The case against bicarbonate therapy. *Ann Intern Med* 1986; **105**:276

Standards for cardiopulmonary resuscitation (CPR) and emergency cardiac care (ECC). *JAMA* 1986; **255**:2905

Weil MH, Rackow EC, Trevino R, *et al.* Difference in acid-base state between venous and arterial blood during cardiopulmonary resuscitation. *N Engl J Med* 1986; **315**:153

Yakaitis RW, Otto CW, Blitt CD. Relative importance of α and β adrenergic receptors during resuscitation. *Crit Care Med* 1979; **7**:293

Notes

3.2 Hypotension

Circulatory management

1. The overall principle in the management of hypotension is to correct to a minimum mean arterial pressure that will maintain tissue perfusion.
2. The circulating volume must be corrected before using catecholamines for hypotension.
3. Most cases of hypotension require fluid as first line management. Exceptions include acute left heart failure, arrhythmias, cardiac tamponade and tension pneumothorax although an adequate circulating volume must be confirmed.
4. Restoration of a normal blood pressure does not guarantee an adequate cardiac output.
5. Cardiac output should usually be measured in patients receiving inotropes.
6. Support of the circulation aims to maintain tissue oxygenation.
   • Increases in cardiac output increase oxygen transport.
   • Increases in blood pressure facilitate perfusion of the microvasculature.

Effects of catecholamines

1. The predominant effects of catecholamines are determined by their receptor activity:

Catecholamine	Predominant receptor(s)	Predominant effects
Dobutamine	β_1	↑↑Stroke volume, ↑Heart rate
Dopamine (low dose)	Dopaminergic	↑Splanchnic and renal perfusion
Adrenaline	β_1, α_1 and β_2	↑Heart rate, ↑Stroke volume, Vasoconstriction
Noradrenaline	α_1	Vasoconstriction
Isoprenaline	β_1 and β_2	↑↑Heart rate, Vasodilatation

2. Dobutamine and isoprenaline may reduce pulmonary vascular resistance.
3. Dobutamine may cause vasodilatation due to β_2 effects.
4. Dobutamine causes less tachycardia than isoprenaline.
5. Tachycardia increases myocardial oxygen demand severely.
6. Critically ill patients, with high circulating levels of endogenous catecholamines, may have down-regulated receptors and may thus require very high doses.

The use of vasopressors in hypotension

1. Vasopressors such as noradrenaline may reduce cardiac output via the increase in peripheral resistance.
2. An adequate cardiac output must be ensured before using vasopressors such as noradrenaline to support the blood pressure.
3. Vasopressors should be used in the smallest dose which achieves an acceptable blood pressure.
4. Although 60 mmHg is a minimum mean arterial pressure to aim for, hypotension is best treated relative to pre-illness values, i.e. a chronic hypertensive may require higher pressures.

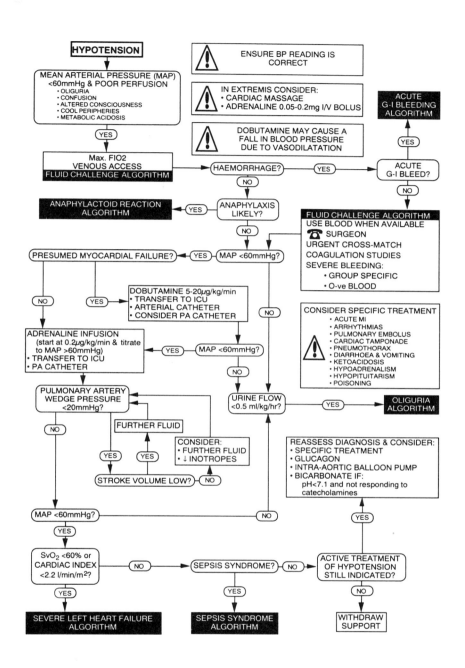

HYPOTENSION

MEAN ARTERIAL PRESSURE (MAP)
<60mmHg & POOR PERFUSION
• OLIGURIA
• CONFUSION
• ALTERED CONSCIOUSNESS
• COOL PERIPHERIES
• METABOLIC ACIDOSIS

⚠ ENSURE BP READING IS CORRECT

⚠ IN EXTREMIS CONSIDER:
• CARDIAC MASSAGE
• ADRENALINE 0.05-0.2mg I/V BOLUS

⚠ DOBUTAMINE MAY CAUSE A FALL IN BLOOD PRESSURE DUE TO VASODILATATION

ACUTE G-I BLEEDING ALGORITHM

YES

Max. FIO2
VENOUS ACCESS
FLUID CHALLENGE ALGORITHM

HAEMORRHAGE? — YES — ACUTE G-I BLEED?

NO

NO

ANAPHYLACTOID REACTION ALGORITHM — YES — ANAPHYLAXIS LIKELY?

NO

FLUID CHALLENGE ALGORITHM
USE BLOOD WHEN AVAILABLE
☎ SURGEON
URGENT CROSS-MATCH
COAGULATION STUDIES
SEVERE BLEEDING:
• GROUP SPECIFIC
• O-ve BLOOD

PRESUMED MYOCARDIAL FAILURE? — YES — MAP <60mmHg?

NO   YES

DOBUTAMINE 5-20µg/kg/min
• TRANSFER TO ICU
• ARTERIAL CATHETER
• CONSIDER PA CATHETER

NO

CONSIDER SPECIFIC TREATMENT
⚠ • ACUTE MI
• ARRHYTHMIAS
• PULMONARY EMBOLUS
• CARDIAC TAMPONADE
• PNEUMOTHORAX
• DIARRHOEA & VOMITING
• KETOACIDOSIS
• HYPOADRENALISM
• HYPOPITUITARISM
• POISONING

ADRENALINE INFUSION
(start at 0.2µg/kg/min & titrate
to MAP >60mmHg)
• TRANSFER TO ICU
• PA CATHETER

YES — MAP <60mmHg?

NO

PULMONARY ARTERY
WEDGE PRESSURE
<20mmHg?

URINE FLOW
<0.5 ml/kg/hr? — YES — OLIGURIA ALGORITHM

NO

FURTHER FLUID

CONSIDER:
• FURTHER FLUID
• ↓ INOTROPES

REASSESS DIAGNOSIS & CONSIDER:
• SPECIFIC TREATMENT
• GLUCAGON
• INTRA-AORTIC BALLOON PUMP
• BICARBONATE IF:
pH<7.1 and not responding to
catecholamines

YES   YES

STROKE VOLUME LOW? — NO

MAP <60mmHg? — NO   YES

YES

SvO2 <60% or
CARDIAC INDEX
<2.2 l/min/m2? — NO — SEPSIS SYNDROME? — NO — ACTIVE TREATMENT OF HYPOTENSION STILL INDICATED?

YES   YES   NO

SEVERE LEFT HEART FAILURE ALGORITHM

SEPSIS SYNDROME ALGORITHM

WITHDRAW SUPPORT

Bibliography

Edwards JD, Brown CS, Nightingale P, *et al.* Use of survivors' cardio-respiratory values as therapeutic goals in septic shock. *Crit Care Med* 1989; **17**:1098

Maekawa K, Liang CS, Hood WB. Comparison of dobutamine and dopamine in acute myocardial infarction. Effects of systemic hemodynamics, plasma catecholamines, blood flows and infarct size. *Circulation* 1983; **67**:750

Meadows D, Edwards JD, Wilkins RG, *et al.* Reversal of intractable septic shock with norepinephrine therapy. *Crit Care Med* 1988; **16**:663

Shoemaker WC, Appel PL, Kram HB, *et al.* Prospective trial of supranormal values of survivors as therapeutic goals in high-risk surgical patients. *Chest* 1988; **94**:1176

Tuttle DR, Pollock GD, Todd G, *et al.* The effect of dobutamine on cardiac oxygen balance, regional blood flow and infarction severity after coronary artery narrowing in dogs. *Circ Res* 1977; **41**:357

Vincent JL, Reuse C, Kahn RJ. Effects on right ventricular function of a change from dopamine to dobutamine in critically ill patients. *Crit Care Med* 1988; **16**:659

Notes

3.3 Severe hypertension

Causes
1. Seek the cause to enable definitive treatment to be given e.g. surgery.
2. Aortic coarctation can present acutely in adults, though usually with heart failure. Check for inequality/absence/delay of pulses.

Management
1. Aim to reduce blood pressure to mildly hypertensive levels, e.g. diastolic 95–110mmHg.
2. If giving I/V infusions, monitor closely, ideally using continuous invasive arterial pressure monitoring.
3. Avoid precipitate drops in BP during therapy as organ perfusion pressures, in particular to the cerebral circulation, may be compromised.
4. Although oral or sublingual nifedipine has been recommended by some authorities, its use may result in unpredictable precipitate drops in BP which may compromise the cerebral circulation leading to strokes, blindness, etc.
5. Sodium nitroprusside is a highly potent antihypertensive; however, cyanide toxicity can develop within 24–48 hours. Therapy should not be continued beyond this period or if an unexplained metabolic acidosis develops.
6. Specific therapy may be indicated for specific conditions e.g. α- and β-blockade for phaeochromocytoma.

Bibliography
Ferguson RK, Vlasses PH. Hypertensive emergencies and urgencies. *JAMA* 1986; **255**: 1607
Komsuoglu SS, Komsuoglu B, Ozmenoglu M, Ozcan C, Gurhan H. Oral nifedipine in the treatment of hypertensive crises in patients with hypertensive encephalopathy. *Int J Cardiol* 1992; **34**: 277
Prisant LM, Carr AA, Hawkins DW. Treating hypertensive emergencies. Controlled reduction of blood pressure and protection of target organs. *Postgrad Med* 1993; **93**: 92

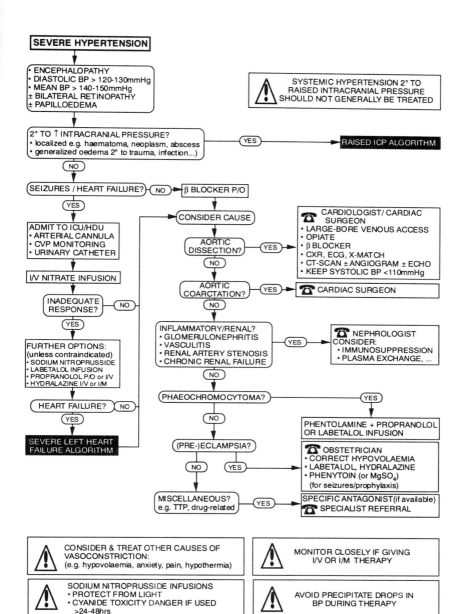

SEVERE HYPERTENSION

- ENCEPHALOPATHY
- DIASTOLIC BP > 120-130mmHg
- MEAN BP > 140-150mmHg
- ± BILATERAL RETINOPATHY
- ± PAPILLOEDEMA

⚠ SYSTEMIC HYPERTENSION 2° TO RAISED INTRACRANIAL PRESSURE SHOULD NOT GENERALLY BE TREATED

2° TO ↑ INTRACRANIAL PRESSURE?
- localized e.g. haematoma, neoplasm, abscess
- generalized oedema 2° to trauma, infection...) —YES→ **RAISED ICP ALGORITHM**

NO

SEIZURES / HEART FAILURE? —NO→ β BLOCKER P/O

YES

ADMIT TO ICU/HDU
- ARTERIAL CANNULA
- CVP MONITORING
- URINARY CATHETER

I/V NITRATE INFUSION

INADEQUATE RESPONSE? —NO→

YES

FURTHER OPTIONS:
(unless contraindicated)
- SODIUM NITROPRUSSIDE
- LABETALOL INFUSION
- PROPRANOLOL P/O or I/V
- HYDRALAZINE I/V or I/M

HEART FAILURE? —NO→

YES

SEVERE LEFT HEART FAILURE ALGORITHM

CONSIDER CAUSE

AORTIC DISSECTION? —YES→ ☎ CARDIOLOGIST/ CARDIAC SURGEON
- LARGE-BORE VENOUS ACCESS
- OPIATE
- β BLOCKER
- CXR, ECG, X-MATCH
- CT-SCAN ± ANGIOGRAM ± ECHO
- KEEP SYSTOLIC BP <110mmHg

NO

AORTIC COARCTATION? —YES→ ☎ CARDIAC SURGEON

NO

INFLAMMATORY/RENAL?
- GLOMERULONEPHRITIS
- VASCULITIS
- RENAL ARTERY STENOSIS
- CHRONIC RENAL FAILURE —YES→ ☎ NEPHROLOGIST
CONSIDER:
- IMMUNOSUPPRESSION
- PLASMA EXCHANGE, ...

NO

PHAEOCHROMOCYTOMA? —YES→

NO

PHENTOLAMINE + PROPRANOLOL OR LABETALOL INFUSION

(PRE-)ECLAMPSIA? ☎ OBSTETRICIAN
- CORRECT HYPOVOLAEMIA
- LABETALOL, HYDRALAZINE
- PHENYTOIN (or $MgSO_4$)
  (for seizures/prophylaxis)

NO   YES

MISCELLANEOUS?
e.g. TTP, drug-related —YES→ SPECIFIC ANTAGONIST(if available)
☎ SPECIALIST REFERRAL

⚠ CONSIDER & TREAT OTHER CAUSES OF VASOCONSTRICTION:
(e.g. hypovolaemia, anxiety, pain, hypothermia)

⚠ MONITOR CLOSELY IF GIVING I/V OR I/M THERAPY

⚠ SODIUM NITROPRUSSIDE INFUSIONS
- PROTECT FROM LIGHT
- CYANIDE TOXICITY DANGER IF USED >24-48hrs

⚠ AVOID PRECIPITATE DROPS IN BP DURING THERAPY

3.4 Acute chest pain

History
1. A careful history is essential. In general:
   - sharp pain affected by breathing—pleuritic (infection/embolus), musculo-skeletal or pericardial in origin
   - dull, continuous pressing pain—myocardial ischaemia/infarction, pneumothorax
   - tender to touch—musculoskeletal (e.g. costochondritis, myalgia, trauma)
   - sharp pain or ache related to meals—peptic, occasionally cardiac
   - pain related to body position—reflux oesophagitis, pericarditis

Management
1. All patients should receive high concentration, high flow oxygen except the small proportion with Type II (chronic hypoxaemic, hypercapnic) respiratory failure [see algorithm 2.5].
2. Thrombolysis has not been shown to be of benefit in unstable angina.
3. Relative contraindications to β-blockade include heart failure, asthma, peripheral vascular disease and diabetes mellitus. Caution should be exercised if used in these conditions.

Analgesia
1. Insufficient or excessive analgesia must be avoided to prevent respiratory compromise. It is very important to remove or minimize pain to allow an adequate depth of inspiration.
2. Consider (unless contraindicated) opiates, simple analgesics, non-steroidals, regional anaesthesia.
3. Opiates should be given in small aliquots e.g. diamorphine 2.5 mg and repeated as indicated.
4. Relative contraindications for the use of non-steroidals include renal dysfunction, peptic ulceration and fluid retention. Caution should be exercised if used in these conditions.

Bibliography
Bar FW, Verhugt F, Col J, *et al.* Thrombolysis in patients with unstable angina improves the angiographic but not the clinical outcome. Results of UNASEM—a multicenter, randomised, placebo-controlled clinical trial with anistreplase. *Circulation* 1992; **86**: 131
DeSanctis RW, Doroghazi RM, Arsten WG, Buckley MJ. Aortic dissection. *N Engl J Med* 1987; **317**: 1060
Editorial: Non-specific chest pain. *Lancet* 1987; **i**: 958
Horgan JH. Cardiac tamponade. *BMJ* 1987; **295**: 563
Johnson PA, Lee TH, Cook EF, Rouan GW, Goldman L. Effect of race on the presentation and management of patients with acute chest pain. *Ann Intern Med* 1993; **118**: 593
TIMI Group. Early effects of tissue type plasminogen activator added to conventional therapy on the culprit lesion in patients presenting with ischemic cardiac pain at rest. Results of the Thrombolysis in Myocardial Ischemia (TIMI IIIA) Trial. *Circulation* 1993; **87**: 38

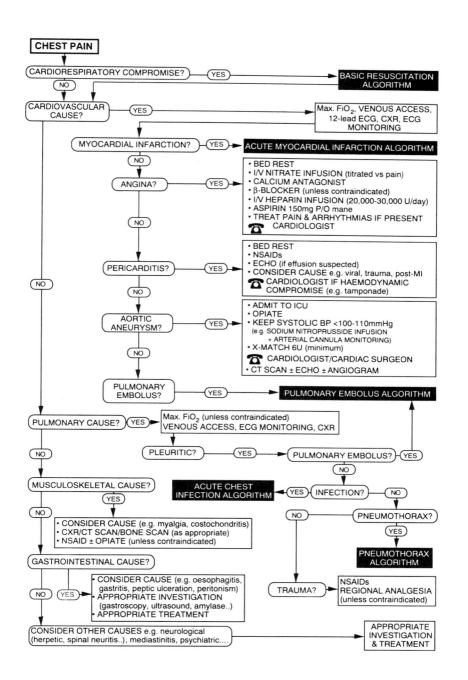

CHEST PAIN

CARDIORESPIRATORY COMPROMISE? — YES → **BASIC RESUSCITATION ALGORITHM**
NO

CARDIOVASCULAR CAUSE? — YES → Max. FiO$_2$, VENOUS ACCESS, 12-lead ECG, CXR, ECG MONITORING
NO

MYOCARDIAL INFARCTION? — YES → **ACUTE MYOCARDIAL INFARCTION ALGORITHM**
NO

ANGINA? — YES →
• BED REST
• I/V NITRATE INFUSION (titrated vs pain)
• CALCIUM ANTAGONIST
• β-BLOCKER (unless contraindicated)
• I/V HEPARIN INFUSION (20,000-30,000 U/day)
• ASPIRIN 150mg P/O mane
• TREAT PAIN & ARRHYTHMIAS IF PRESENT
☎ CARDIOLOGIST
NO

PERICARDITIS? — YES →
• BED REST
• NSAIDs
• ECHO (if effusion suspected)
• CONSIDER CAUSE e.g. viral, trauma, post-MI
☎ CARDIOLOGIST IF HAEMODYNAMIC COMPROMISE (e.g. tamponade)
NO

AORTIC ANEURYSM? — YES →
• ADMIT TO ICU
• OPIATE
• KEEP SYSTOLIC BP <100-110mmHg
  (e.g. SODIUM NITROPRUSSIDE INFUSION
   + ARTERIAL CANNULA MONITORING)
• X-MATCH 6U (minimum)
☎ CARDIOLOGIST/CARDIAC SURGEON
• CT SCAN ± ECHO ± ANGIOGRAM
NO

PULMONARY EMBOLUS? — YES → **PULMONARY EMBOLUS ALGORITHM**

PULMONARY CAUSE? — YES → Max. FiO$_2$ (unless contraindicated) VENOUS ACCESS, ECG MONITORING, CXR
NO

PLEURITIC? — YES → PULMONARY EMBOLUS? — YES
NO

INFECTION? — YES → **ACUTE CHEST INFECTION ALGORITHM**
NO

MUSCULOSKELETAL CAUSE? — YES →
NO

• CONSIDER CAUSE (e.g. myalgia, costochondritis)
• CXR/CT SCAN/BONE SCAN (as appropriate)
• NSAID ± OPIATE (unless contraindicated)

PNEUMOTHORAX? — YES → **PNEUMOTHORAX ALGORITHM**
NO

TRAUMA? → NSAIDs REGIONAL ANALGESIA (unless contraindicated)

GASTROINTESTINAL CAUSE?
NO   YES →
• CONSIDER CAUSE (e.g. oesophagitis, gastritis, peptic ulceration, peritonism)
• APPROPRIATE INVESTIGATION (gastroscopy, ultrasound, amylase..)
• APPROPRIATE TREATMENT

CONSIDER OTHER CAUSES e.g. neurological (herpetic, spinal neuritis..), mediastinitis, psychiatric.... → **APPROPRIATE INVESTIGATION & TREATMENT**

3.5 Acute myocardial infarction

Thrombolysis
1. Effective up to 24 hrs. Give preferably within 4–6 hrs from onset of symptoms.
2. Revascularization arrhythmias are common post-thrombolysis. Of these over 90% are benign and do not require treatment.
3. Contraindications to thrombolysis:

Absolute contraindications	Relative contraindications
active G-I bleeding	traumatic or prolonged CPR
aortic dissection	recent obstetric delivery
neurosurgery/head injury/CVA within 2 months	prior organ biopsy
intracranial neoplasm/aneurysm	
proliferative diabetic retinopathy	bleeding diathesis
serious trauma, major surgery within 10 days	(recent puncture of major vessel)
systolic BP >200 mmHg	

3. Streptokinase is the current first-line therapy unless the patient has had a previous reaction to it, has received it within the previous 5 days to 54 months, has had a recent streptococcal infection (< 1 month), or if an imminent surgical or invasive procedure is anticipated. If so, use tissue plasminogen activator (rTPA) which can also be considered as first-line therapy in young patients (<45 years), in large anterior MI presenting early (<4 hrs), and in cardiogenic shock.
4. rTPA should not be used more than 6 hours after onset of symptoms (except when streptokinase previously given), in patients over 75 years old, and in the absence of diagnostic ECG changes.
5. Arterial and/or central venous cannulation should not be delayed if clinically indicated. It should be performed by an experienced operator, *avoiding* the subclavian route.
6. Thrombolysis may be given even when relative contraindications exist, when the mortality risk from MI (e.g. with associated hypotension) outweighs the risk of bleeding.
7. Allergic reactions to thrombolytic therapy should be treated:
   • stop streptokinase
   • hydrocortisone 100 mg I/V
   • chlorpheniramine 10 mg I/V
   • ranitidine 50 mg I/V
   • give rTPA instead
8. If severe bleeding occurs during thrombolysis, or urgent surgery is required:
   • stop infusion
   • give aprotonin 500,000 units over 10 min, then 200,000 units over 4 hrs
   • OR give tranexamic acid 10 mg/kg repeated after 6–8 hrs
   • FFP (though must give with aprotonin or tranexamic acid)
9. Hypotension:
   • prior to thrombolysis?   rTPA preferable
   • during/after thrombolysis? Reduce/temporarily stop; support circulation and aim to continue
10. There is no added benefit to aspirin by giving heparin.
11. I/V heparin should be used after rTPA (proven benefit). It should also be considered for large infarcts and heart failure.

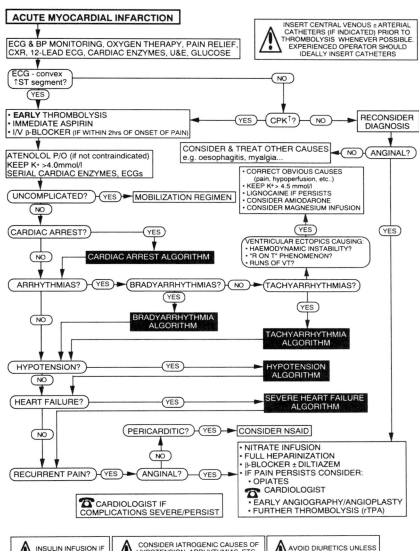
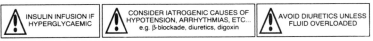

Drug doses

1. Diamorphine — 2.5 mg I/V. Repeat prn + anti-emetic
2. Streptokinase — 1.5 million units in 100 ml 0.9% saline I/V over 1 hr
3. rTPA — 100 mg I/V over 90 min(15 mg bolus, 50 mg/30 min, 35 mg/60 min)
4. APSAC — 30 units I/V over 5 min
5. Aspirin — 150 mg P/O od
6. Atenolol — 50 mg P/O od (increase to100 mg od if not hypotensive & HR >70 bpm)
7. Propranolol — 10–40 mg P/O qid (titrate to HR of 60 bpm)
8. Isosorbide dinitrate — 2–40 mg/hr I/V
9. GTN — 10–200 µg/min I/V
10. Diltiazem — 60 mg P/O tid
11. Nifedipine — 5–10 mg S/L or P/O tid
12. Atropine — 0.3 mg I/V. Repeated to maximum of 2 mg
13. Isoprenaline — 1–4 µg/min. Titrate to clinical effect.
14. Lignocaine — 1 mg/kg I/V bolus then 2–4 mg/min (1% solution contains 10 mg/ml)
15. Amiodarone — 5 mg/kg over 15 min then infused up to 15 mg/kg/day in 5% glucose via central vein
(In emergency:150–300 mg in 10-20 ml 5% glucose over 1–2 min)
16. Magnesium — $MgSO_4$ 8 mmol over 20 mins then 65 mmol over 24 hrs

Diagnosis

1. Approximately 20% of patients with subsequently proved infarction will present without ST elevation or clearly identifiable Q waves. Perform repeated ECG/CPK if in doubt.
2. A rise in CPK to diagnostic levels (×2 normal) may take up to 4–8 hrs.

Complications

1. Any suspicion of a low output state should result in active treatment. Early consideration should be given to placement of a pulmonary artery catheter.
2. An early cardiological opinion should be sought in patients with low output states as balloon angioplasty or early surgery may improve the prognosis in this high-risk group. Early angioplasty following thrombolysis has not been shown to be of benefit in asymptomatic patients but may be useful as an alternative, or in selected patients.
3. Hypotension may be iatrogenic, e.g. excessive diuretics, β-blockers.
4. Rarer causes of post-infarction heart failure and low output states should be considered, e.g. VSD, chordal rupture.
5. Patients developing post-infarction ventricular failure should be commenced on ACE inhibitors; this does however await large study confirmation.
6. When anginal-type pain persists post-infarction and does not settle on medical therapy, early angiography ± angioplasty ± early bypass grafting should be considered. Neither surgical technique will enhance resting ventricular function though it may prevent further deterioration.

Management

1. Diuretics are rarely needed if the patient does not have fluid overload or chronic heart failure. They may increase cardiac work by vasoconstriction secondary to volume depletion and activation of the renin-angiotensin-aldosterone system.

2. Low dose nitrate infusions will cause hypotension in the underfilled patient.
3. Right ventricular infarction may result in left ventricular underfilling. Fluid loading and/or inotropes are then indicated and a pulmonary artery catheter should be considered for precise management.
4. Unless contraindicated, atenolol 5 mg I/V may be given within 2 hrs of onset of pain
5. Caution should be exercised when giving non-steroidal anti-inflammatory drugs such as indomethacin as this may result in fluid retention.
6. Calcium antagonists have been shown to be of no overall value post-infarction.

Bibliography

AIMS trial study group. Effect of intravenous APSAC on mortality after acute myocardial infarction: preliminary report of a placebo-controlled trial. *Lancet* 1988; **i**: 545

Caplin JL. Acute right ventricular infarction. *BMJ* 1989; **299**: 459

Chatterjee K, Swan HJC, Kaushik VS, *et al.* Effects of vasodilator therapy for severe pump failure in acute myocardial infarction on short-term and late prognosis. *Circulation* 1976; **53**: 797

Chesebro JH, Knatterud G, Roberts R, *et al.* Thrombolysis in myocardial infarction (TIMI) trial, Phase I: a comparison between intravenous tissue plasminogen activator and intravenous streptokinase. *Circulation* 1987; **76**: 142

Gruppo Italiano per lo studio della streptochinasi nell'infarcto miocardico (GISSI). Effectiveness of intravenous thrombolytic treatment in acute myocardial infarction. *Lancet* 1986; **i**: 397

Gruppo Italiano per lo studio della streptochinasi nell'infarcto miocardico. GISSI-2. A factorial randomised trial of alteplase versus streptokinase and heparin versus no heparin among 12490 patients with acute myocardial infarction. *Lancet* 1990; **336**: 65

Randomised trial of intravenous streptokinase, oral aspirin, both, or neither among 17187 cases of suspected acute myocardial infarction: ISIS-2. *Lancet* 1988; **ii**: 349

The GUSTO Investigators. An international randomised trial comparing four thrombolytic strategies for acute myocardial infarction. *N Engl J Med* 1993; **329**: 673

Johnson SA, Scanlon PJ, Loeb HS, Moran JM, Pifarre R, Gunnar RM. Treatment of cardiogenic shock in myocardial infarction by intra-aortic balloon counterpulsation and surgery. *Am J Med* 1977; **62**: 687

Teo KK, Yusuf S, Collins R, Held PH, Peto R. Effects of intravenous magnesium in suspected acute myocardial infarction. Overview of randomised trials. *BMJ* 1991; **303**: 1499

Lee L, Bates ER, Pitt B, Walton JA, Laufer N, O'Neill WW. Percutaneous transluminal coronary angioplasty improves survival in acute myocardial infarction complicated by cardiogenic shock. *Circulation* 1988; **78**: 1345

Pfeffer MA, Braunwald E, Moyle LA, *et al.* Effect of captopril on mortality and morbidity in patients with left ventricular dysfunction after myocardial infarction. *N Engl J Med* 1992; **327**: 669

Swedberg K, Held P, *et al.* Effects of the early administration of enalapril on mortality in patients with acute myocardial infarction. Results of the cooperative new Scandinavian enalapril survival study II (CONSENSUS II). *N Engl J Med* 1992; **327**: 678

Yusuf S, Peto R, Lewis J, Collins R, Sleight P. Beta-blockade during and after myocardial infarction: an overview of the randomised trials. *Prog Cardiovasc Dis* 1985; **27**: 335

3.6/3.7 Bradyarrhythmia/Tachyarrhythmia

General management of bradyarrhythmia
1. Treat if there is (impending) haemodynamic compromise or disturbance of cerebral function.
2. Treat the cause of the arrhythmia whenever possible.
3. Bradycardia and/or heart block occurring acutely after an inferior MI are often short-lived, requiring atropine only. If pacing is necessary normal sinus rhythm is usually regained by 7–10 days.
4. Higher degrees of heart block often require permanent pacing.
5. Sino-atrial disorders usually require permanent pacing.

Indications for temporary pacing in bradyarrhythmia
1. Persistence of symptomatic bradycardia.
2. Blackouts associated with
   - 3° heart block
   - 2° heart block
   - RBBB and Left posterior hemiblock
3. Cardiovascular failure.
4. Inferior MI with 3° heart block.
5. Anterior MI with
   - 3° heart block
   - RBBB and Left posterior hemiblock
   - alternating RBBB and LBBB

General management of tachyarrhythmia
1. Treat if there is (impending) haemodynamic compromise.
2. Treat the cause of the arrhythmia whenever possible.
3. Amiodarone and magnesium sulphate are useful for most tachyarrhythmias.
4. Drugs used for chronic treatment of arrhythmias may not be appropriate acutely.
5. Many patients requiring antiarrhythmic therapy acutely will not require long term therapy.
6. The risks of digitalis toxicity are higher in critically ill patients with poor hepatic or renal function.
7. Pacing should be available prior to treatment of digoxin-induced tachyarrhythmias.
8. Cardioversion in digoxin toxicity may cause dangerous arrhythmias.
9. Unsuccessful digitalis therapy increases the risks of side-effects from other antiarrhythmic therapy.

Management of atrial and supraventricular tachyarrhythmias
1. Atrial flutter with 2:1 block should be suspected in any regular narrow complex tachycardia at 130–160/min.
2. Adenosine has a very rapid onset of action and a short half life. Incremental doses can be repeated in quick succession.
3. Adenosine can be used in Wolff–Parkinson–White syndrome though the rate may increase.
4. Adenosine will not convert atrial fibrillation or flutter to sinus rhythm but may slow the rate.
5. Adenosine should not be used for sick sinus syndrome.
6. Verapamil has a rapid onset of action and a fairly short duration. Incremental doses should not be given within 10 minutes of the last dose.

7. Hypotension with verapamil usually responds to intravenous calcium.
8. Hypotension with amiodarone is often secondary to the solvent and is avoided by slow intravenous bolus injection.
9. The use of verapamil is contraindicated if the patient is β blocked.

Management of ventricular tachyarrhythmias

1. The use of verapamil in misdiagnosed ventricular tachycardia may cause life-threatening hypotension.
2. Intravenous amiodarone can successfully revert otherwise intractable ventricular tachycardia.
3. Amiodarone can be used in combination with other therapy for ventricular tachycardia (although not with sotalol since both have class III activity and would severely prolong the QT interval).
4. Overpacing is indicated if a pacind wire is in situ or if drug therapy fails.
5. Torsades de pointes may be aggravated by antiarrhythmic therapy. Treatment includes reversal of the underlying cause, $MgSO_4$ and isoprenaline in cases where Torsades follows a bradyarrhythmia.

Antiarrhythmic drug dosages

1. Atropine   0.3 mg I/V. Repeated as necessary to maximum of 2.1 mg
2. Isoprenaline $1-10$ µg/min
3. Adenosine   3 mg I/V. If no response in 1 min give 6 mg I/V followed by 12 mg I/V
4. Verapamil   2.5 mg I/V. Repeated as necessary to maximum of 20 mg. Consider I/V infusion of $1-10$ mg/hr
5. Lignocaine   1 mg/kg I/V bolus then $2-4$ mg/min (1% solution contains 10 mg/ml)
6. Amiodarone   5 mg/kg over 15 min then infused up to 15 mg/kg/day in 5% glucose via central vein (In emergency: $150-300$ mg in $10-20$ ml 5% glucose over $1-2$ min)
7. Magnesium $MgSO_4$ 20 mmol over $2-3$ hr

Bibliography

Aronow WS, Aronow W. Clinical use of digitalis. *Compr Ther* 1992; **18**:38
Faniel R, Schoenfeld Ph. Efficacy of iv amiodarone in converting rapid atrial fibrillation and atrial flutter to sinus rhythm in intensive care patients. *Eur Heart J* 1983; **4**:180
Iberti TJ, Benjamin E, Paluch TA, *et al.* Use of constant infusion verapamil for the treatment of postoperative supraventricular tachycardia. *Crit Care Med* 1986; **14**:283
Kastor JA. Atrioventricular block. *N Engl J Med* 1975; **462**:572
Munoz A, Karila P, Gallay P, Zettelmeier F, Messner P, Mery M, Grolleau R. A randomized hemodynamic comparison of intravenous amiodarone with and without Tween 80. *Eur Heart J* 1988; **9**:142
Reiter MJ, Shand DG, Aanonsen LM, *et al.* Pharmacokinetics of verapamil: Experience with a sustained intravenous infusion regimen. *Am J Cardiol* 1982; **50**:716
Saksena S, Kesselbrenner MB. Current perspectives in management of ventricular tachyarrhythmias with intravenous and oral amiodarone. *Clin Prog Electrophysiol Pacing* 1986; **4**:382
Sung RJ, Shapiro WA, Shen EN, *et al.* Effects of verapamil on ventricular tachycardias possibly caused by re-entry, automaticity and triggered activity. *J Clin Invest* 1983; **72**:350
Wyse DG. Pharmacologic therapy in patients with ventricular tachyarrhythmias. *Cardiol Clin* 1993; **11**:65

CARDIOVASCULAR

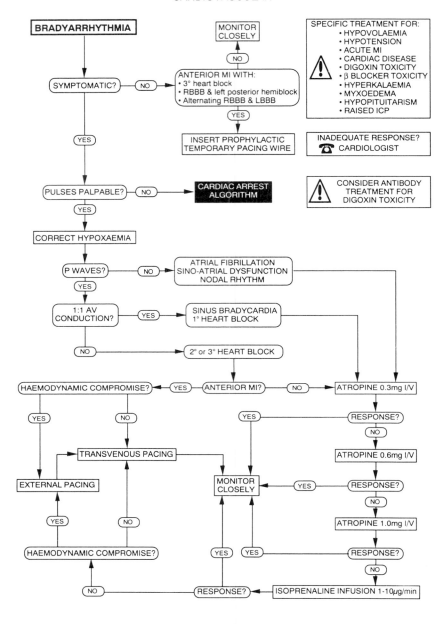

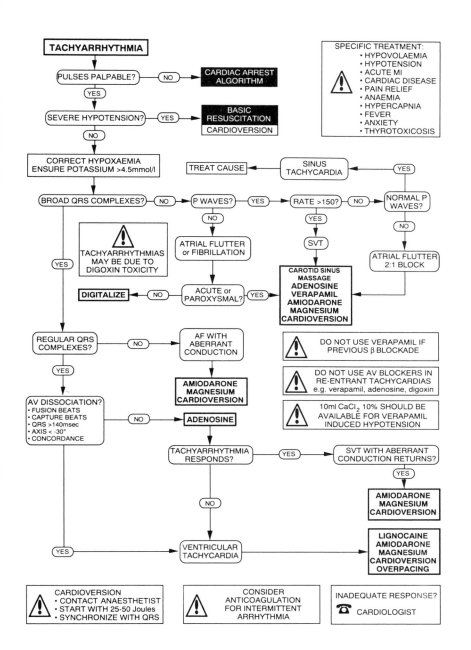

TACHYARRHYTHMIA

PULSES PALPABLE? —NO→ CARDIAC ARREST ALGORITHM

YES

SEVERE HYPOTENSION? —YES→ BASIC RESUSCITATION / CARDIOVERSION

NO

CORRECT HYPOXAEMIA ENSURE POTASSIUM >4.5mmol/l

SPECIFIC TREATMENT:
- HYPOVOLAEMIA
- HYPOTENSION
- ACUTE MI
- CARDIAC DISEASE
- PAIN RELIEF
- ANAEMIA
- HYPERCAPNIA
- FEVER
- ANXIETY
- THYROTOXICOSIS

TREAT CAUSE ←— SINUS TACHYCARDIA ←—YES—

BROAD QRS COMPLEXES? —NO→ P WAVES? —YES→ RATE >150? —NO→ NORMAL P WAVES?

YES (P WAVES?) NO

NO (RATE >150?) YES → SVT

NO (NORMAL P WAVES?) → ATRIAL FLUTTER 2:1 BLOCK

TACHYARRHYTHMIAS MAY BE DUE TO DIGOXIN TOXICITY

ATRIAL FLUTTER or FIBRILLATION

CAROTID SINUS MASSAGE ADENOSINE VERAPAMIL AMIODARONE MAGNESIUM CARDIOVERSION

DIGITALIZE ←NO— ACUTE or PAROXYSMAL? —YES→

YES

REGULAR QRS COMPLEXES? —NO→ AF WITH ABERRANT CONDUCTION

YES

AMIODARONE MAGNESIUM CARDIOVERSION

DO NOT USE VERAPAMIL IF PREVIOUS β BLOCKADE

DO NOT USE AV BLOCKERS IN RE-ENTRANT TACHYCARDIAS e.g. verapamil, adenosine, digoxin

10ml CaCl₂ 10% SHOULD BE AVAILABLE FOR VERAPAMIL INDUCED HYPOTENSION

AV DISSOCIATION?
- FUSION BEATS
- CAPTURE BEATS
- QRS >140msec
- AXIS < -30°
- CONCORDANCE

—NO→ ADENOSINE

TACHYARRHYTHMIA RESPONDS? —YES→ SVT WITH ABERRANT CONDUCTION RETURNS?

YES

AMIODARONE MAGNESIUM CARDIOVERSION

NO

YES→ VENTRICULAR TACHYCARDIA →

LIGNOCAINE AMIODARONE MAGNESIUM CARDIOVERSION OVERPACING

CARDIOVERSION
- CONTACT ANAESTHETIST
- START WITH 25-50 Joules
- SYNCHRONIZE WITH QRS

CONSIDER ANTICOAGULATION FOR INTERMITTENT ARRHYTHMIA

INADEQUATE RESPONSE?
☎ CARDIOLOGIST

3.8 Severe left heart failure

Respiratory management
1. High concentration high flow oxygen therapy is mandatory.
2. Early ventilation should be considered in severe cardiac failure:
   * reduced work of breathing
   * reduced metabolic rate
   * diaphragmatic failure associated with inadequate cardiac output
   * reduced cardiac distension due to reduced venous return
   * allows the use of sedatives and anxiolytics
   * reduced left ventricular afterload
3. CPAP usually improves gas exchange in severe pulmonary oedema but should not be allowed to reduce cardiac output.

Fluid and diuretic management
1. Caution should be exercised in the use of frusemide.
2. Patients rarely die of pulmonary oedema in heart failure; rather they die of organ hypoperfusion.
3. Pulmonary oedema does *not* indicate total body fluid overload. It may take days for the lymphatics to achieve radiological clearing.
4. Peripheral oedema does usually suggest salt and water retention. Diuretics may be appropriate in this situation though caution should be exercised as intravascular fluid depletion may also co-exist.
5. Fluid overload is not usually a feature of acute heart failure; fluid is maldistributed so excessive diuresis should be avoided.
6. Cardiac performance in severe heart failure is worsened by compensatory vasoconstriction. Diuretics will cause further vasoconstriction by hypovolaemia.
7. Any beneficial effects of frusemide in acute heart failure without fluid overload are due to early and transient venodilatation.
8. Oliguria may be due to hypovolaemia (sweating, vomiting, not drinking, diuretics) rather than cardiogenic pump failure.

Peripheral circulatory management
1. Nitrates produce an improved cardiac performance in severe heart failure by:
   * decreased peripheral resistance
   * reduced cardiac distension by reduced venous return
   * possibly increased coronary perfusion
2. Hypotension is not a problem with nitrates if cardiac filling pressures are maintained.
3. A drop in BP following low dose nitrates or ACE inhibitors suggests hypovolaemia.
4. Normalizing a raised SVR is an important method of improving cardiac efficiency.

Catecholamines
1. Catecholamines should be used sparingly in acute heart failure since they increase myocardial oxygen demand and decrease myocardial cAMP.
2. Inotropic catecholamines should not be titrated against blood pressure; rather they should be titrated against measures of adequacy of the circulation:
   * mixed venous oxygen saturation(SvO_2)>60%
   * normal blood lactate
   * cardiac index >2.2 l/min/m^2

3. Vasopressor catecholamines are usually not required in acute heart failure since peripheral resistance is usually high.
4. Phosphodiesterase inhibitors may restore catecholamine sensitivity by reducing cAMP depletion.

Monitoring

1. The CVP is a poor guide to left heart filling pressures in either right or left heart failure.
2. Both the CVP and PAWP poorly reflect end-diastolic ventricular volumes due to changes in ventricular compliance.
3. A PAWP of 15–18 mmHg is usually adequate but may need to be higher in chronic cardiac failure. However, because of changes in ventricular compliance, a dynamic fluid (or nitrate) challenge is the best means of assessing volaemic status [see Algorithm 1.1].
4. A fall in SvO_2 is the earliest indicator of circulatory inadequacy.

Bibliography

Aubier M, Trippenbach T, Roussos C. Respiratory muscle fatigue during cardiogenic shock. *J Appl Physiol* 1981; **51**:499

Baratz DM, Westbrook PR, Shah PK, Mohsenifar Z. Effect of nasal continuous positive airway pressure on cardiac output and oxygen delivery in patients with congestive heart failure. *Chest* 1992; **102**: 1397

Bussman W, Schupp D. Effect of sublingual nitroglycerin in emergency treatment of severe pulmonary edema. *Am J Cardiol* 1978; **41**:931

Creamer J, Edwards JD, Nightingale P. Haemodynamic and oxygen transport variables in cardiogenic shock following acute myocardial infarction and their response to treatment. *Am J Cardiol* 1990; **65**:1297

Dikshit K, Vyden JK, Forrester JS, Chatterjee K, Prakash R, Swan HJC. Renal and extrarenal hemodynamic effects of furosemide in congestive heart failure after acute myocardial infarction. *N Engl J Med* 1973; **288**:1087

Forrester JS, Diamond G, McHugh T, Swan HJC. Filling pressures in the right and left sides of the heart in acute myocardial infarction. A reappraisal of central venous pressure monitoring. *N Engl J Med* 1971; **285**:190

Nelson GIC, Ahuja RC, Silke B, Hussain M, Taylor SH. Haemodynamic advantages of isosorbide dinitrate over frusemide in acute heart failure following myocardial infarction. *Lancet* 1983; **i**:730

Nelson GIC, Silke B, Forsyth DR, Verma SP, Hussain M, Taylor SH. Hemodynamic comparison of primary venous or arteriolar dilatation and the subsequent effect of furosemide in left ventricular failure after acute myocardial infarction. *Am J Cardiol* 1983; **52**:1036

Singer M, Bennett ED. Intravenous nitrates in severe left ventricular failure with hypotension. *Crit Care Med* 1989; **17**:S134

Singer M. The management of acute heart failure: an iconoclastic view. *Care of the Critically Ill* 1993; **9**: 11

CARDIOVASCULAR

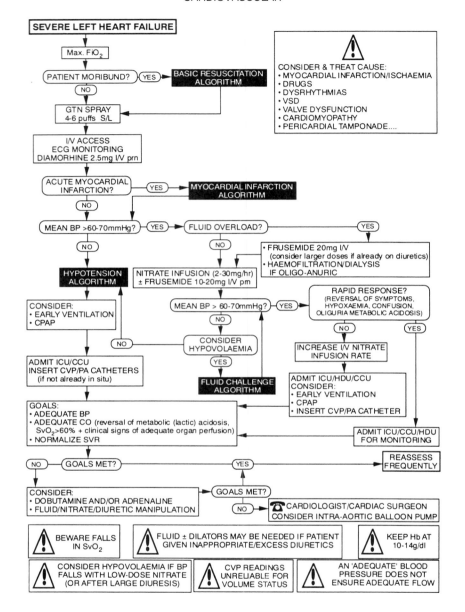

SEVERE LEFT HEART FAILURE

Max. FiO$_2$

PATIENT MORIBUND? — YES → **BASIC RESUSCITATION ALGORITHM**

NO

GTN SPRAY
4-6 puffs S/L

I/V ACCESS
ECG MONITORING
DIAMORHINE 2.5mg I/V prn

ACUTE MYOCARDIAL INFARCTION? — YES → **MYOCARDIAL INFARCTION ALGORITHM**

NO

MEAN BP >60-70mmHg? — YES → FLUID OVERLOAD? — YES

NO

NO

⚠ CONSIDER & TREAT CAUSE:
• MYOCARDIAL INFARCTION/ISCHAEMIA
• DRUGS
• DYSRHYTHMIAS
• VSD
• VALVE DYSFUNCTION
• CARDIOMYOPATHY
• PERICARDIAL TAMPONADE....

HYPOTENSION ALGORITHM

NITRATE INFUSION (2-30mg/hr)
± FRUSEMIDE 10-20mg I/V prn

• FRUSEMIDE 20mg I/V
(consider larger doses if already on diuretics)
• HAEMOFILTRATION/DIALYSIS
IF OLIGO-ANURIC

CONSIDER:
• EARLY VENTILATION
• CPAP

MEAN BP > 60-70mmHg? — YES

NO

RAPID RESPONSE?
(REVERSAL OF SYMPTOMS,
HYPOXAEMIA, CONFUSION,
OLIGURIA METABOLIC ACIDOSIS)

NO → INCREASE I/V NITRATE INFUSION RATE

YES

NO → CONSIDER HYPOVOLAEMIA

YES

ADMIT ICU/CCU
INSERT CVP/PA CATHETERS
(if not already in situ)

FLUID CHALLENGE ALGORITHM

ADMIT ICU/HDU/CCU
CONSIDER:
• EARLY VENTILATION
• CPAP
• INSERT CVP/PA CATHETER

GOALS:
• ADEQUATE BP
• ADEQUATE CO (reversal of metabolic (lactic) acidosis,
SvO$_2$>60% + clinical signs of adequate organ perfusion)
• NORMALIZE SVR

ADMIT ICU/CCU/HDU
FOR MONITORING

NO — GOALS MET? — YES → REASSESS FREQUENTLY

CONSIDER:
• DOBUTAMINE AND/OR ADRENALINE
• FLUID/NITRATE/DIURETIC MANIPULATION

GOALS MET?

NO → ☎ CARDIOLOGIST/CARDIAC SURGEON
CONSIDER INTRA-AORTIC BALLOON PUMP

⚠ BEWARE FALLS IN SvO$_2$

⚠ FLUID ± DILATORS MAY BE NEEDED IF PATIENT GIVEN INAPPROPRIATE/EXCESS DIURETICS

⚠ KEEP Hb AT 10-14g/dl

⚠ CONSIDER HYPOVOLAEMIA IF BP FALLS WITH LOW-DOSE NITRATE (OR AFTER LARGE DIURESIS)

⚠ CVP READINGS UNRELIABLE FOR VOLUME STATUS

⚠ AN 'ADEQUATE' BLOOD PRESSURE DOES NOT ENSURE ADEQUATE FLOW

Notes

3.9 Pulmonary embolus

Diagnosis

1. Suspect when:
   - acute dyspnoea, ± pleuritic pain, ± haemoptysis, ± low BP, raised JVP, syncope, cyanosis
   - pulmonary oligaemia on chest X-ray
   - ECG changes (S_1,Q_3,T_3, right axis deviation, right bundle branch block, tachycardia.)
   - blood gas changes (low PaO_2, low $PaCO_2$, metabolic acidosis)
   - ± clinical history of DVT
2. A radioisotope ventilation-perfusion scan will provide an indication of the likelihood of PE.
3. A normal plasma D-dimer level is a good means of excluding pulmonary embolus.
4. An abnormal pulmonary angiogram provides the definitive diagnosis.

Treatment

1. The role of surgery is controversial. It may be of benefit for single, centrally-placed, massive clots.
2. Fluid loading is the important first step in circulatory management and should be given before inotropes.
3. The patient may prefer to lie flat and dyspnoea may improve.
4. Gas exchange may worsen with mechanical ventilation because of loss of preferential shunting.

Thrombolysis

1. Early thrombolytic therapy is important.
2. No comparative trials have studied large bolus doses of streptokinase.
3. Thrombolysis with rTPA followed by heparin anticoagulation is superior to heparin alone.

Bibliography

Editorial: Thrombolysis for pulmonary embolus. *Lancet* 1992; **340**:21
Goldhaber SZ, Kessler CM, Heit J, *et al*. Randomised controlled trial of recombinant tissue plasminogen activator vs urokinase in the treatment of acute pulmonary embolus. *Lancet* 1988; **i**: 293
Goldhaber SZ, Haire WD, Feldstein ML, *et al*. Alteplase versus heparin in acute pulmonary embolism: randomised trial assessing right ventricular function and pulmonary perfusion. *Lancet* 1993; **341**: 507
Goldhaber SZ, Simons GR, Elliott G, *et al*. Quantitative plasma D-Dimer levels among patients undergoing pulmonary angiography for suspected pulmonary embolism. *JAMA* 1993; 2819
Gray HH, Firoozan S. The pulmonary physician and critical care. 5. Management of pulmonary embolism. *Thorax* 1992; **47**: 825
Harrison KA, Haire WD, Pappas AA, *et al*. Plasma D-dimer: a useful tool for evaluating suspected pulmonary embolus. *J Nucl Med* 1993; **34**: 896
Meyer G, Surs H, Charbonnier B, *et al*. Effects of intraveous urokinase versus alteplase on total pulmonary resistance in acute massive pulmonary embolism: a European multicenter double-blind trial. *J Am Coll Cardiol* 1992; **19**: 239
Stein PD, Hull RD, Saltzman HA, Pineo G. Strategy for diagnosis of patients with suspected acute pulmonary embolism. *Chest* 1993; **103**: 1553

PULMONARY EMBOLUS

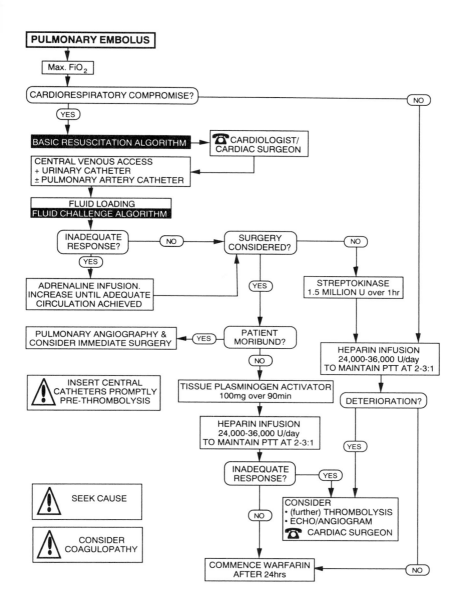

Max. FiO$_2$

CARDIORESPIRATORY COMPROMISE? ─────────────────────────── NO

YES

BASIC RESUSCITATION ALGORITHM ──→ ☎ CARDIOLOGIST/ CARDIAC SURGEON

CENTRAL VENOUS ACCESS
+ URINARY CATHETER
± PULMONARY ARTERY CATHETER

FLUID LOADING
FLUID CHALLENGE ALGORITHM

INADEQUATE RESPONSE? ── NO ── SURGERY CONSIDERED? ── NO

YES

ADRENALINE INFUSION.
INCREASE UNTIL ADEQUATE
CIRCULATION ACHIEVED

YES

STREPTOKINASE
1.5 MILLION U over 1hr

PULMONARY ANGIOGRAPHY &
CONSIDER IMMEDIATE SURGERY ── YES ── PATIENT MORIBUND?

NO

HEPARIN INFUSION
24,000-36,000 U/day
TO MAINTAIN PTT AT 2-3:1

⚠ INSERT CENTRAL
CATHETERS PROMPTLY
PRE-THROMBOLYSIS

TISSUE PLASMINOGEN ACTIVATOR
100mg over 90min

DETERIORATION?

HEPARIN INFUSION
24,000-36,000 U/day
TO MAINTAIN PTT AT 2-3:1

YES

INADEQUATE RESPONSE? ── YES

⚠ SEEK CAUSE

CONSIDER
• (further) THROMBOLYSIS
• ECHO/ANGIOGRAM
☎ CARDIAC SURGEON

NO

⚠ CONSIDER
COAGULOPATHY

COMMENCE WARFARIN
AFTER 24hrs ←──────────── NO

4. Renal

4.1/4.2 Oliguria/acute renal failure

Urinary tract obstruction
1. Exclude a blocked catheter (common).
2. An ultrasound is suitable to exclude obstruction.
3. An intravenous urogram may be hazardous in renal failure due to nephrotoxic contrast.

Urinalysis
1. It is mandatory to test for protein, sugar and blood.
2. Red cell casts indicate glomerular disease.
3. WBC (infection) and crystals (obstruction) may provide useful diagnostic information.

Chemistry
1. A low urinary sodium (<20 mmol/l) suggests hypovolaemia. It may be spuriously high after diuretics. It may be misleadingly low in urinary tract obstruction or hepatorenal syndrome.
2. Differentiation of hypovolaemia from parenchymal renal failure:

	Hypovolaemia (pre-renal)	Renal
urine osmolality (mOsm/kg)	>500	<400
urinary Na	<20	>40
urine:plasma creatinine	>40	<20
fractional excretion Na^+ (%)	<1 $100\times \dfrac{\text{urine:plasma } Na^+}{\text{urine:plasma creatinine}}$	>2

3. In practice, the important steps are to exclude obstruction, correct hypovolaemia and hypotension, and treat the cause. Chemical ratios are rarely needed.

Diagnosing the cause of established renal failure
1. Many drugs are potentially nephrotoxic in a variety of ways:
   - acute tubular necrosis
   - interstitial nephritis
   - renal tubular obstruction
2. Drugs must be withheld during the diagnostic period if at all possible.
3. Consider rhabdomyolysis and myoglobinuria in oliguric patients, particularly if unconscious (e.g. from overdose) or involved in crush injury. Measure plasma CPK, urinary myoglobin. Creatinine is very high compared to urea.
4. Urgent assistance from a nephrologist is required in diagnosis of established renal failure; a renal biopsy is usually required.
5. Immunosuppressive treatment may salvage adequate renal function but should only be started on the advice of a nephrologist.

Treatment aims in established renal failure
1. Treatment should remove reversible causes of acute renal failure and correct metabolic abnormalities arising as a consequence of renal failure.
2. Plasma urea and creatinine are a guide to treatment; they are not in themselves toxic.

3. Prevention of hyperkalaemia and metabolic acidosis is necessary to prevent fatal cardiac arrhythmias.
4. Fluid management aims at correcting reversible pre-renal failure and at the same time avoiding fluid overload.

Treatment

1. Correct hypovolaemia before giving drugs.
2. Diuretics may have a place in prophylaxis in some situations. Not shown to affect rate of recovery of established acute renal failure.
3. There is only limited evidence of the value of dopamine as prophylaxis against renal failure in man. There is no convincing evidence of its value in established renal failure.
4. Drug dosages should be modified in acute renal failure, n.b.
   • antibiotics (aminoglycosides, penicillins...)
   • sedatives
   • muscle relaxants
   • digoxin
5. Bigger doses of diuretics may be needed in long-term diuretic takers.
6. Failure to re-establish urine flow makes transfer to a dialysis unit inevitable.
7. If anuria persists, remove urinary catheter.
8. Acute renal failure patients are usually catabolic; adequate nutrition must be provided.

Bibliography

Amerio A, Corabelli P, Campese VM, et al. Acute renal failure. Advances in experimental medicine and biology Vol. 212. Plenum Press, New York, London, 1986

Aronoff GR. Nonsteroidal anti-inflammatory drug induced renal syndromes. J Ky Med Assoc 1992; 90:336

Miller TR. Urinary diagnostic indices in acute renal failure: a prospective study. Ann Intern Med 1978; 89:47

Prichard BN, Owens CW, Woolf AS. Adverse reactions to diuretics. Eur Heart J 1992; 13 (Suppl G):96

Schrier RW. Renal and electrolyte disorders. 3rd edition. Little Brown, Boston, Toronto, 1986

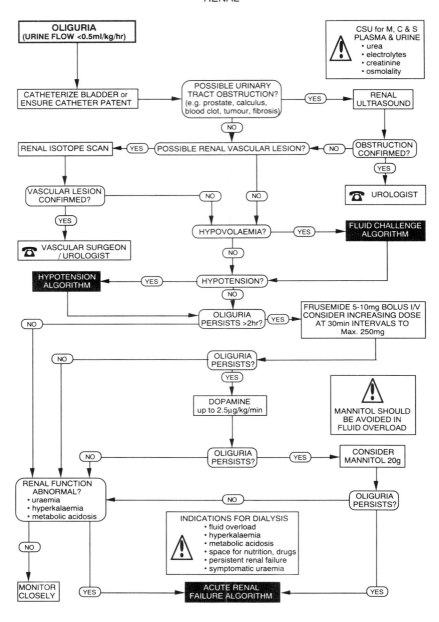

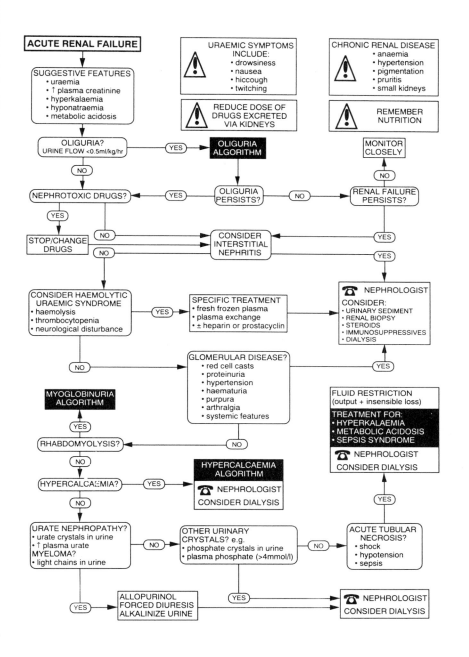

ACUTE RENAL FAILURE

SUGGESTIVE FEATURES
• uraemia
• ↑ plasma creatinine
• hyperkalaemia
• hyponatraemia
• metabolic acidosis

URAEMIC SYMPTOMS
INCLUDE:
• drowsiness
• nausea
• hiccough
• twitching

REDUCE DOSE OF
DRUGS EXCRETED
VIA KIDNEYS

CHRONIC RENAL DISEASE
• anaemia
• hypertension
• pigmentation
• pruritis
• small kidneys

REMEMBER
NUTRITION

OLIGURIA?
URINE FLOW <0.5ml/kg/hr — YES → OLIGURIA
ALGORITHM

MONITOR
CLOSELY

NO

NEPHROTOXIC DRUGS? ← YES — OLIGURIA
PERSISTS? — NO → RENAL FAILURE
PERSISTS?

NO

YES

STOP/CHANGE
DRUGS

NO

NO

CONSIDER
INTERSTITIAL
NEPHRITIS ← YES

YES

YES

CONSIDER HAEMOLYTIC
URAEMIC SYNDROME
• haemolysis
• thrombocytopenia
• neurological disturbance — YES →

SPECIFIC TREATMENT
• fresh frozen plasma
• plasma exchange
• ± heparin or prostacyclin

☎ NEPHROLOGIST
CONSIDER:
• URINARY SEDIMENT
• RENAL BIOPSY
• STEROIDS
• IMMUNOSUPPRESSIVES
• DIALYSIS

NO

GLOMERULAR DISEASE?
• red cell casts
• proteinuria
• hypertension
• haematuria
• purpura
• arthralgia
• systemic features — YES

**MYOGLOBINURIA
ALGORITHM**

YES

RHABDOMYOLYSIS? ← NO

NO

FLUID RESTRICTION
(output + insensible loss)

TREATMENT FOR:
• HYPERKALAEMIA
• METABOLIC ACIDOSIS
• SEPSIS SYNDROME

☎ NEPHROLOGIST
CONSIDER DIALYSIS

HYPERCALCAEMIA? — YES →

**HYPERCALCAEMIA
ALGORITHM**

☎ NEPHROLOGIST
CONSIDER DIALYSIS

NO

YES

URATE NEPHROPATHY?
• urate crystals in urine
• ↑ plasma urate
MYELOMA?
• light chains in urine — NO →

OTHER URINARY
CRYSTALS? e.g.
• phosphate crystals in urine
• plasma phosphate (>4mmol/l) — NO →

ACUTE TUBULAR
NECROSIS?
• shock
• hypotension
• sepsis

YES

ALLOPURINOL
FORCED DIURESIS
ALKALINIZE URINE — YES →

☎ NEPHROLOGIST
CONSIDER DIALYSIS

4.3. Myoglobinuria/haemoglobinuria/haematuria

Rhabdomyolysis

1. Causes
   - trauma/crush injury
   - vascular occlusion (post-vascular surgery)
   - prolonged immobilization
   - drugs e.g. opiates, Ecstasy
   - burns, electrocution
   - hyperpyrexia
   - infection
2. Suspect from history or if plasma creatinine is disproportionately high compared to urea.
3. The urine need not be obviously coloured for significant rhabdomyolysis to be present.
4. Hypocalcaemia and hyperphosphataemia should only be treated if symptomatic; however, hypomagnesaemia should be corrected.
5. Adequate rehydration and a good diuresis are crucial in preventing renal failure. Alkalinization of the urine (pH $\geq$6) aids urinary excretion of myoglobin.
6. Hyperkalaemia may be very resistant to standard treatment. Urgent dialysis may be needed.

Compartment syndrome

1. Perform fasciotomies when compartment pressures > 25 mmHg or if a high risk exists for developing compression.
2. Loss of peripheral pulses and leg swelling are relatively late signs. Earlier indicators include pain and cold peripheries.
3. Beware potential large blood loss with fasciotomies.

Intravascular haemolysis

1. Causes
   - malaria
   - drugs
   - sickle cell crisis, thalassaemia, G6PD deficiency
   - immune (Rhesus, warm or cold Ab)
   - hypersplenism
   - cardiac valve prosthesis

Haematuria

1. Causes
   - trauma/foreign body
   - haemolytic uraemic syndrome
   - glomerulonephritis (red cell casts)
   - Berger's disease
   - neoplasm

Bibliography

Better OS, Stein JH. Early management of shock and prophylaxis of acute renal failure in traumatic rhabdomyolysis. *N Engl J Med* 1990; **322**: 825
Gabow PA, Kaehry WD, Kelleher SP. The spectrum of rhabdomyolysis. *Medicine* 1982; **61**:141
Tabbara IA. Hemolytic anemias. Diagnosis and management. *Med Clin North Am* 1992; **76**: 649

MYOGLOBINURIA/HAEMOGLOBINURIA/HAEMATURIA

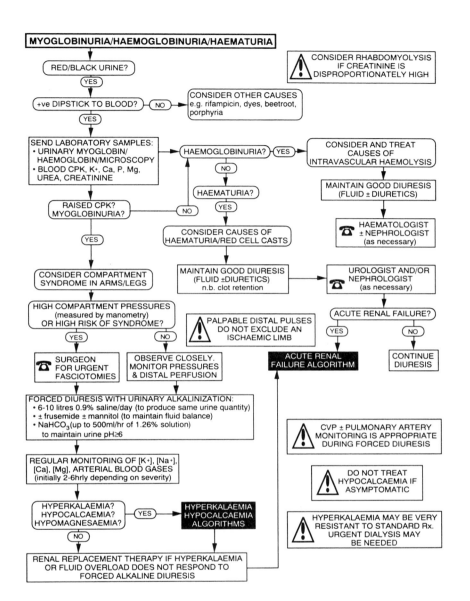

RED/BLACK URINE?

⚠ CONSIDER RHABDOMYOLYSIS IF CREATININE IS DISPROPORTIONATELY HIGH

YES

+ve DIPSTICK TO BLOOD? → NO → CONSIDER OTHER CAUSES e.g. rifampicin, dyes, beetroot, porphyria

YES

SEND LABORATORY SAMPLES:
• URINARY MYOGLOBIN/ HAEMOGLOBIN/MICROSCOPY
• BLOOD CPK, K+, Ca, P, Mg, UREA, CREATININE

HAEMOGLOBINURIA? → YES → CONSIDER AND TREAT CAUSES OF INTRAVASCULAR HAEMOLYSIS

NO

HAEMATURIA?

MAINTAIN GOOD DIURESIS (FLUID ± DIURETICS)

RAISED CPK? MYOGLOBINURIA? → NO

YES

☎ HAEMATOLOGIST ± NEPHROLOGIST (as necessary)

CONSIDER CAUSES OF HAEMATURIA/RED CELL CASTS

CONSIDER COMPARTMENT SYNDROME IN ARMS/LEGS

MAINTAIN GOOD DIURESIS (FLUID ±DIURETICS) n.b. clot retention

☎ UROLOGIST AND/OR NEPHROLOGIST (as necessary)

HIGH COMPARTMENT PRESSURES (measured by manometry) OR HIGH RISK OF SYNDROME?

⚠ PALPABLE DISTAL PULSES DO NOT EXCLUDE AN ISCHAEMIC LIMB

ACUTE RENAL FAILURE?

YES   NO

YES   NO

☎ SURGEON FOR URGENT FASCIOTOMIES

OBSERVE CLOSELY. MONITOR PRESSURES & DISTAL PERFUSION

ACUTE RENAL FAILURE ALGORITHM

CONTINUE DIURESIS

FORCED DIURESIS WITH URINARY ALKALINIZATION:
• 6-10 litres 0.9% saline/day (to produce same urine quantity)
• ± frusemide ± mannitol (to maintain fluid balance)
• NaHCO$_3$(up to 500ml/hr of 1.26% solution) to maintain urine pH≥6

⚠ CVP ± PULMONARY ARTERY MONITORING IS APPROPRIATE DURING FORCED DIURESIS

REGULAR MONITORING OF [K+], [Na+], [Ca], [Mg], ARTERIAL BLOOD GASES (initially 2-6hrly depending on severity)

⚠ DO NOT TREAT HYPOCALCAEMIA IF ASYMPTOMATIC

HYPERKALAEMIA? HYPOCALCAEMIA? HYPOMAGNESAEMIA? → YES → HYPERKALAEMIA HYPOCALCAEMIA ALGORITHMS

⚠ HYPERKALAEMIA MAY BE VERY RESISTANT TO STANDARD Rx. URGENT DIALYSIS MAY BE NEEDED

NO

RENAL REPLACEMENT THERAPY IF HYPERKALAEMIA OR FLUID OVERLOAD DOES NOT RESPOND TO FORCED ALKALINE DIURESIS

5. Metabolic

5.1 Hypernatraemia

1. Symptoms include thirst, lethargy, coma, convulsions, muscular tremor and rigidity, and an increased risk of intracranial haemorrhage.
2. Treatment depends upon the cause and whether there is normal, low or elevated total body sodium stores and normal or low body water.
3. Aim for gradual correction of plasma Na (over 1–3 days), particularly in chronic cases (>2 days' duration), to avoid cerebral oedema through sudden lowering of osmolality.
4. If hypernatraemia is accompanied by haemodynamic alterations secondary to hypovolaemia, colloid (or isotonic saline) should be used initially to restore the circulation.
5. Artificial colloid solutions consist of starches (e.g. Hespan) or gelatins (e.g. Gelofusin, Haemaccel) dissolved in isotonic saline.
6. Thirst usually occurs when the plasma sodium rises 3–4 mmol/l above normal. Lack of thirst is associated with CNS disease.

Type	Aetiology	Urine
LOW TOTAL BODY Na	RENAL LOSSES osmotic diuretics (glucose, urea, mannitol)	$[Na^+]$ >20 mmol/l iso- or hypotonic
	EXTRA-RENAL LOSSES excess sweating, diarrhoea in children	$[Na^+]$ <10 mmol/l hypertonic
NORMAL TOTAL BODY Na	RENAL LOSSES nephrogenic diabetes insipidus central diabetes insipidus hypodipsia	$[Na^+]$ variable hypo-, iso- or hypertonic
	EXTRA-RENAL LOSSES respiratory and dermal insensible losses	$[Na^+]$ variable hypertonic
INCREASED TOTAL BODY Na	Conn's syndrome, Cushing's syndrome, hypertonic sodium bicarbonate, sodium chloride tablets	$[Na^+]$ > 20 mmol/l iso- or hypertonic

Diabetes insipidus (DI)

1. Cranial DI may be complete or partial. Salt restriction and thiazide diuretics are useful for both. Complete cranial DI will require dDAVP whereas partial cranial DI may require dDAVP but will often respond to drugs that increase the rate of ADH secretion or end-organ responsiveness to ADH e.g. chlorpropamide, hydrochlorthiazide.
2. Nephrogenic DI should also be managed by a low salt diet and thiazides. dDAVP may be necessary. Consider removal of causative agents e.g. lithium, demeclocycline.

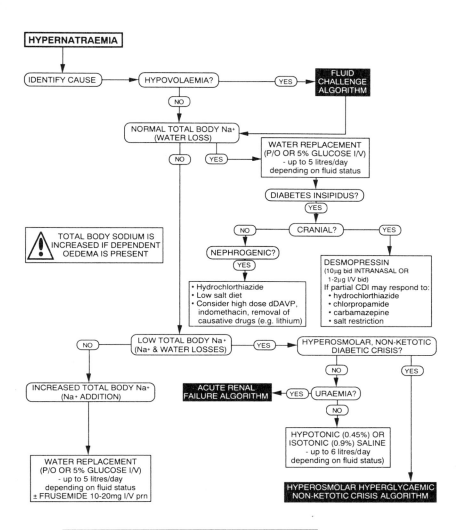

HYPERNATRAEMIA

IDENTIFY CAUSE → HYPOVOLAEMIA? → YES → **FLUID CHALLENGE ALGORITHM**

NO

NORMAL TOTAL BODY Na+ (WATER LOSS)

NO   YES → WATER REPLACEMENT (P/O OR 5% GLUCOSE I/V) - up to 5 litres/day depending on fluid status

DIABETES INSIPIDUS?

YES

NO → CRANIAL? → YES

NEPHROGENIC?

YES

⚠ TOTAL BODY SODIUM IS INCREASED IF DEPENDENT OEDEMA IS PRESENT

- Hydrochlorthiazide
- Low salt diet
- Consider high dose dDAVP, indomethacin, removal of causative drugs (e.g. lithium)

DESMOPRESSIN
(10µg bid INTRANASAL OR 1-2µg I/V bid)
If partial CDI may respond to:
- hydrochlorthiazide
- chlorpropamide
- carbamazepine
- salt restriction

NO   LOW TOTAL BODY Na+ (Na+ & WATER LOSSES) → YES → HYPEROSMOLAR, NON-KETOTIC DIABETIC CRISIS?

NO   YES

INCREASED TOTAL BODY Na+ (Na+ ADDITION)

ACUTE RENAL FAILURE ALGORITHM ← YES ← URAEMIA?

NO

HYPOTONIC (0.45%) OR ISOTONIC (0.9%) SALINE - up to 6 litres/day depending on fluid status)

WATER REPLACEMENT (P/O OR 5% GLUCOSE I/V) - up to 5 litres/day depending on fluid status ± FRUSEMIDE 10-20mg I/V prn

HYPEROSMOLAR HYPERGLYCAEMIC NON-KETOTIC CRISIS ALGORITHM

⚠ CORRECTION RATE:
HYPERACUTE HYPERNATRAEMIA (<12hr): CAN BE RAPID
CHRONIC HYPERNATRAEMIA (>2 days): <0.7mmol/l/hr

Bibliography

Berl T, Anderson RJ, McDonald KM, Scrier RW. Clinical disorders of water metabolism. *Kidney Int* 1976; **10**:117

Oh MS, Carroll HJ. Disorders of sodium metabolism: Hypernatremia and hyponatremia. *Crit Care Med* 1992; **20**:94

Rose BD. New approach to disturbances in the plasma sodium concentration. *Am J Med* 1986; **81**: 1033

Notes

5.2 Hyponatraemia

1. Symptoms—nausea, vomiting, headache, fatigue, weakness, muscular twitching, obtundation, psychosis, convulsions and coma—depend on rate as well as magnitude of fall in [Na] level.
2. In chronic hyponatraemia correction should not exceed 0.5 mmol/l/hr in the first 24 hr and 0.3 mmol/l/hr thereafter.
3. In acute hyponatraemia the ideal rate of correction is controversial. It is generally agreed that elevations in plasma sodium level can be faster, but no greater than 20 mmol/l/day.
   If doubt exists as to speed of onset of hyponatraemia, treat as if acute hyponatraemia.
4. A plasma sodium level of 125–130 mmol/l is a reasonable target to aim for in initial correction of both acute and chronic states. Attempts to rapidly achieve normo- or hypernatraemia should be avoided. Neurological complications e.g. central pontine myelinolysis, osmotic demyelination syndrome are related to the degree of correction and (in chronic hyponatraemia) the rate. Women are more prone to these complications.
5. Equations that calculate excess water are unreliable. It is safer to perform frequent estimations of plasma sodium levels.
6. Hypertonic saline infusions may be dangerous in the elderly or those with impaired cardiac function. An alternative is to use frusemide with replacement of urinary sodium (and potassium) losses each 2–3 hr. Thereafter simple water restriction is usually sufficient.
   n.b. many patients achieve normonatraemia by spontaneous water diuresis.
7. Use isotonic solutions for reconstituting drugs, parenteral nutrition, bladder irrigation, etc.
8. Severe hyponatraemia has been corrected safely by haemofiltration.
9. Hyponatraemia may intensify the cardiac effects of hyperkalaemia.
10. Spurious hyponatraemia may be due to (i) 'drip' artefacts if taken from same arm as a running infusion. (n.b. serum osmolality is not reduced by an appropriate extent) or (ii) analytical artefacts—hyperproteinaemia or hypertriglyceridaemia if using flame photometry or 'indirect' ion-specific electrodes (ISE). 'Direct-reading' ISEs are not susceptible to these changes in plasma water content though are sensitive to interference by excess heparin.
11. A true hyponatraemia may occur with a normal osmolality in the presence of abnormal solutes e.g. methanol, ethanol, ethylene glycol, glucose, mannitol.

Type	Aetiology	Urinary [Na+]
ECF VOLUME DEPLETION	RENAL LOSSES diuretic excess, mineralocorticoid deficiency, salt-losing nephritis, renal tubular acidosis, osmotic diuresis (glucose, urea, mannitol)	>20 mmol/l
	EXTRA-RENAL LOSSES vomiting, diarrhoea, burns, pancreatitis	<10 mmol/l

Type	Aetiology	Urinary [Na+]
MODEST ECF VOLUME EXCESS (NO OEDEMA)	water intoxication (n.b. post-operative, TURP), inappropriate ADH secretion, glucocorticoid deficiency, hypothyroidism, drugs (e.g. chlorpropamide, carbamazepine), pain, emotion...	>20 mmol/l
ECF VOLUME EXCESS (OEDEMA)	acute and chronic renal failure	>20 mmol/l
	nephrotic syndrome, cirrhosis, cardiac failure	<10 mmol/l

Causes of inappropriate ADH secretion

- neoplasm e.g. lung, pancreas, lymphoma
- most pulmonary lesions
- most CNS lesions
- surgical and emotional stress
- glucocorticoid and thyroid deficiency
- idiopathic
- drugs e.g. chlorpropamide, carbamazepine, narcotics

Bibliography

Arieff AI. Hyponatremia, convulsions, respiratory arrest, and permanent brain damage after elective surgery in healthy women. *N Engl J Med* 1986; **314**: 1529

Arieff AI. Management of hyponatraemia. *BMJ* 1993; **307**: 305

Ayus JC, Olivero JJ, Frommer JP. Rapid correction of severe hyponatraemia with intravenous hypertonic saline solution. *Am J Med* 1982; **72**: 43

Berl T, Anderson RJ, McDonald KM, Schrier RW. Clinical disorders of water metabolism. *Kidney Int* 1976; **10**:117

Cluitmans FHM, Meinders AE. Management of severe hyponatremia: Rapid or slow correction? *Am J Med* 1990; **88**: 161

Foote JW. Hyponatraemia: Diagnosis and management. *Hosp Update* 1990; **12**: 248

Larner AJ, Vickers CR, Adu D, Buchles JAC, Elias E, Neuberger J. Correction of severe hyponatraemia by continuous arteriovenous haemofiltration before liver transplantation. *BMJ* 1988; **297**: 1514

Laureno R, Karp BI. Pontine and extra-pontine myelinolysis following rapid correction of hyponatraemia. *Lancet* 1988; **i**:1439

Oh MS, Carroll HJ. Disorders of sodium metabolism: Hypernatremia and hyponatremia. *Crit Care Med* 1992; **20**:94

Rossi NF. Crucial and practical aspects in the therapy of hyponatremia. *Intensive & Crit Care Digest* 1989; **8**: 35

Sterns RH, Riggs JE, Schochet SS. Osmotic demyelination syndrome following correction of hyponatremia. *N Engl J Med* 1986; **314**: 1535

Sterns RH. Severe symptomatic hyponatraemia: Treatment and outcome. A study of 64 cases. *Ann Intern Med* 1987; **107**: 656

Sterns RH, Thomas DJ, Herndon RM. Brain dehydration and neurologic deterioration after rapid correction of hyponatraemia. *Kidney Int* 1989; **35**: 69

Sterns RH. The treatment of hyponatraemia: first, do no harm. *Am J Med* 1990; **88**: 557

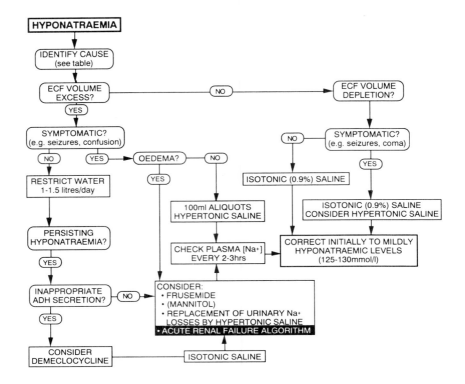

HYPONATRAEMIA

IDENTIFY CAUSE
(see table)

ECF VOLUME EXCESS? ——NO——→ ECF VOLUME DEPLETION?

YES

SYMPTOMATIC?
(e.g. seizures, confusion)

SYMPTOMATIC?
(e.g. seizures, coma)

NO ——— YES — OEDEMA? — NO

NO ——

YES

RESTRICT WATER
1-1.5 litres/day

YES

ISOTONIC (0.9%) SALINE

100ml ALIQUOTS
HYPERTONIC SALINE

ISOTONIC (0.9%) SALINE
CONSIDER HYPERTONIC SALINE

PERSISTING
HYPONATRAEMIA?

CHECK PLASMA [Na+]
EVERY 2-3hrs

CORRECT INITIALLY TO MILDLY
HYPONATRAEMIC LEVELS
(125-130mmol/l)

YES

INAPPROPRIATE
ADH SECRETION? ——NO——

CONSIDER:
• FRUSEMIDE
• (MANNITOL)
• REPLACEMENT OF URINARY Na+
LOSSES BY HYPERTONIC SALINE
• ACUTE RENAL FAILURE ALGORITHM

YES

CONSIDER
DEMECLOCYCLINE ———— ISOTONIC SALINE

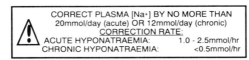

⚠ CORRECT PLASMA [Na+] BY NO MORE THAN
20mmol/day (acute) OR 12mmol/day (chronic)
CORRECTION RATE:
ACUTE HYPONATRAEMIA: 1.0 - 2.5mmol/hr
CHRONIC HYPONATRAEMIA: <0.5mmol/hr

 CARE WITH HYPERTONIC SOLUTIONS:
• n.b. ELDERLY, CARDIAC DYSFUNCTION
• CHECK [Na+] LEVELS 2-3hrly
• CONSIDER PA CATHETER INSERTION

⚠ OVERDIURESIS CAN CAUSE
HYPONATRAEMIA AND
INTRAVASCULAR FLUID DEPLETION
DESPITE PRESENCE OF OEDEMA

 APPROPRIATE SPECIFIC THERAPY
e.g. • steroids for hypoadrenalism
• discontinue diuretic therapy
• discontinue drugs impairing water excretion

⚠ CORRECT COINCIDENT POTASSIUM
AND MAGNESIUM LOSSES

Notes

5.3/5.4 Hyperkalaemia/hypokalaemia

General physiology
1. Intracellular potassium accounts for 98% of total body potassium at a concentration of about 160 mmol/l.
2. Plasma potassium depends on the balance between intake, excretion and the distribution of potassium across cell membranes.
3. Potassium excretion is normally controlled by the kidneys.

Hyperkalaemia
1. Hyperkalaemia is less common than hypokalaemia but more dangerous.
2. Symptoms are poorly correlated to the degree of hyperkalaemia.
3. Clinical symptoms usually occur after ECG changes.
4. Total body potassium is usually not raised significantly in hyperkalaemia.
5. Hyperkalaemia may be associated with total body potassium depletion if there is a coincident metabolic acidosis.
6. The effects of glucose and insulin on potassium levels occur within 30 min and last 1–2 hr.
7. The effects of calcium on hyperkalaemia are rapid but short-lived.
8. Calcium Resonium should be started promptly.

Hypokalaemia
1. Hypokalaemia is not always associated with potassium depletion.
2. Clinical symptoms are usually well correlated with the degree of hypokalaemia, the degree of any associated potassium depletion and the rate at which hypokalaemia develops.
3. Arrhythmias may occur with hypokalaemia and no potassium depletion but most clinical features are associated with severe potassium depletion.
4. Potassium depletion is usually associated with metabolic alkalosis due to increased renal H^+ excretion, particularly if there is co-existent sodium depletion.
5. Hypokalaemia may be associated with metabolic acidosis in renal tubular acidosis, diabetic ketoacidosis, near drowning in fresh water and with a ureterocolic conduit.
6. If hypokalaemia is associated with metabolic acidosis potassium deficiency is severe.
7. Chronic hypokalaemia is associated with vacuolation of renal tubular cells.
8. Potassium infusion should not exceed 30–40 mmol/hr or 200 mmol/day.

Bibliography
Gill JR. Bartter's syndrome. *Ann Rev Med* 1980; **31**:405
Haffner CA, Kendall MJ. Metabolic effects of beta 2-agonists. *J Clin Pharm Ther* 1992; **17**:155
Isaac G, Holland OB. Drug-induced hypokalaemia. A cause for concern. *Drugs Ageing* 1992; **2**:35
Kunan RT, Stein JH. Disorders of hypo- and hyperkalaemia. *Clin Nephrol* 1977; **7**:173
Millane TA, Ward DE, Camm AJ. Is hypomagnesemia arrhythmogenic? *Clin Cardiol* 1992; **15**:103
Prichard BN, Owens CW, Woolf AS. Adverse reactions to diuretics. *Eur Heart J* 1992; **13** (Suppl G):96

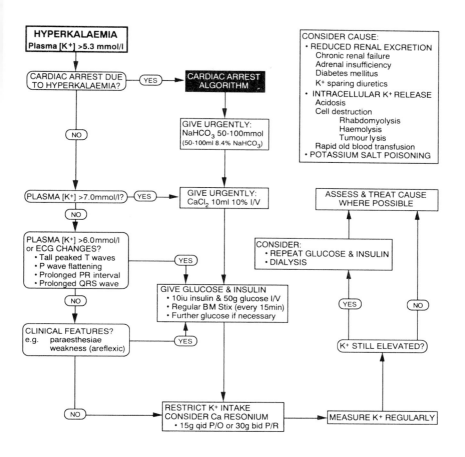

HYPERKALAEMIA
Plasma [K⁺] >5.3 mmol/l

CARDIAC ARREST DUE TO HYPERKALAEMIA? — YES → **CARDIAC ARREST ALGORITHM**

NO

GIVE URGENTLY:
NaHCO₃ 50-100mmol
(50-100ml 8.4% NaHCO₃)

PLASMA [K⁺] >7.0mmol/l? — YES → GIVE URGENTLY:
CaCl₂ 10ml 10% I/V

NO

PLASMA [K⁺] >6.0mmol/l
or ECG CHANGES?
• Tall peaked T waves
• P wave flattening
• Prolonged PR interval
• Prolonged QRS wave

YES

NO

CLINICAL FEATURES?
e.g.   paraesthesiae
       weakness (areflexic)

YES

NO

GIVE GLUCOSE & INSULIN
• 10iu insulin & 50g glucose I/V
• Regular BM Stix (every 15min)
• Further glucose if necessary

RESTRICT K⁺ INTAKE
CONSIDER Ca RESONIUM
• 15g qid P/O or 30g bid P/R

MEASURE K⁺ REGULARLY

K⁺ STILL ELEVATED?

YES   NO

CONSIDER:
• REPEAT GLUCOSE & INSULIN
• DIALYSIS

ASSESS & TREAT CAUSE WHERE POSSIBLE

CONSIDER CAUSE:
• REDUCED RENAL EXCRETION
  Chronic renal failure
  Adrenal insufficiency
  Diabetes mellitus
  K⁺ sparing diuretics
• INTRACELLULAR K⁺ RELEASE
  Acidosis
  Cell destruction
      Rhabdomyolysis
      Haemolysis
      Tumour lysis
  Rapid old blood transfusion
• POTASSIUM SALT POISONING

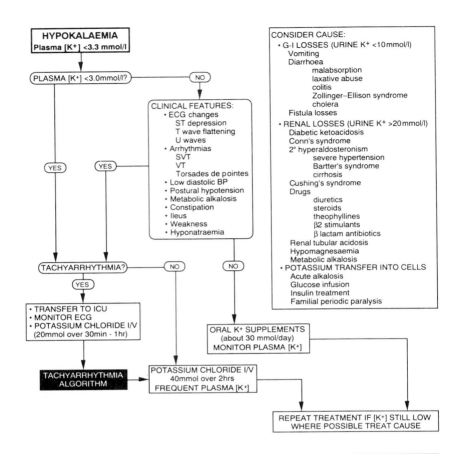

HYPOKALAEMIA
Plasma [K⁺] <3.3 mmol/l

PLASMA [K⁺] <3.0mmol/l? — NO

CLINICAL FEATURES:
- ECG changes
  ST depression
  T wave flattening
  U waves
- Arrhythmias
  SVT
  VT
  Torsades de pointes
- Low diastolic BP
- Postural hypotension
- Metabolic alkalosis
- Constipation
- Ileus
- Weakness
- Hyponatraemia

CONSIDER CAUSE:
- G-I LOSSES (URINE K⁺ <10mmol/l)
  Vomiting
  Diarrhoea
      malabsorption
      laxative abuse
      colitis
      Zollinger–Ellison syndrome
      cholera
  Fistula losses
- RENAL LOSSES (URINE K⁺ >20mmol/l)
  Diabetic ketoacidosis
  Conn's syndrome
  2° hyperaldosteronism
      severe hypertension
      Bartter's syndrome
      cirrhosis
  Cushing's syndrome
  Drugs
      diuretics
      steroids
      theophyllines
      β2 stimulants
      β lactam antibiotics
  Renal tubular acidosis
  Hypomagnesaemia
  Metabolic alkalosis
- POTASSIUM TRANSFER INTO CELLS
  Acute alkalosis
  Glucose infusion
  Insulin treatment
  Familial periodic paralysis

YES   YES

TACHYARRHYTHMIA? — NO   NO

YES

- TRANSFER TO ICU
- MONITOR ECG
- POTASSIUM CHLORIDE I/V
  (20mmol over 30min - 1hr)

ORAL K⁺ SUPPLEMENTS
(about 30 mmol/day)
MONITOR PLASMA [K⁺]

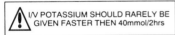

POTASSIUM CHLORIDE I/V
40mmol over 2hrs
FREQUENT PLASMA [K⁺]

REPEAT TREATMENT IF [K⁺] STILL LOW
WHERE POSSIBLE TREAT CAUSE

⚠ I/V POTASSIUM SHOULD RARELY BE
GIVEN FASTER THEN 40mmol/2hrs

⚠ DIGOXIN POTENTIATED BY LOW [K⁺]
WITHHOLD UNTIL [K⁺] CORRECTED

Notes

5.5 Hypercalcaemia

1. Symptoms include nausea, vomiting, abdominal pain, constipation, polyuria, depression, weight loss, fatigue, impaired conscious level, renal calculi, renal failure, arrhythmias, acute pancreatitits.
2. Symptoms depend on age, duration and rate of increase of plasma calcium, and presence of concurrent medical conditions.
3. Causes include:
   • malignancy (e.g. myeloma, metastases...)
   • hyperparathyroidism
   • sarcoidosis
   • vitamin A and D overdose
   • drugs including thiazides, lithium
   • immobilization

Management

1. Rehydration often lowers plasma calcium by 0.4–0.6 mmol/l and should precede diuretics or any other form of treatment.
2. Dialysis/haemofiltration is however indicated if the patient is in established oligoanuric renal failure ± fluid overloaded.
3. Steroids may be effective for haematological cancers (lymphoma, myeloma), vitamin D overdose and sarcoidosis. A 3–5 day course is given.
4. Diphosphonates (e.g. etridonate), mithramycin and especially I/V phosphate should only be given after specialist advice is taken in view of their toxicity and potential complications.
5. Calcitonin has the most rapid onset of action with a nadir often reached within 12–24 hrs. Its action is usually short-lived and rebound hypercalcaemia may occur. It generally does not drop the plasma level by more than 0.5 mmol/l.

Diuretics

1. Frusemide increases calciuria by inhibiting calcium reabsorption in the ascending limb of the loop of Henle.
2. Do not use thiazides which enhance tubular reabsorption and may indeed precipitate hypercalcaemia.
3. More aggressive frusemide regimes e.g. 80–100 mg I/V 1–2 hrly can be used effectively but are more problematic—careful monitoring and attention to fluid balance is mandatory.

Bibliography

Bilezikian J. Management of acute hypercalcaemia. *N Engl J Med* 1992; **326**: 1196
Hosking DJ, Cowley A, Ducknall CA. Rehydration in the treatment of severe hypercalcaemia. *Q J Med* 1981; **50**: 473
Ralston SH. Medical management of hypercalcaemia. *Br J Clin Pharmacol* 1992; **34**: 11
Rizzoli R, Bonjour JP. Management of disorders of calcium homeostasis. *Ballieres Clin Endocrinol Metab* 1992; **6**: 129
Suki WN, Yium JJ, Von Minden M, *et al.* Acute treatment of hypercalcaemia with furosemide. *N Engl J Med* 1970; **283**: 836

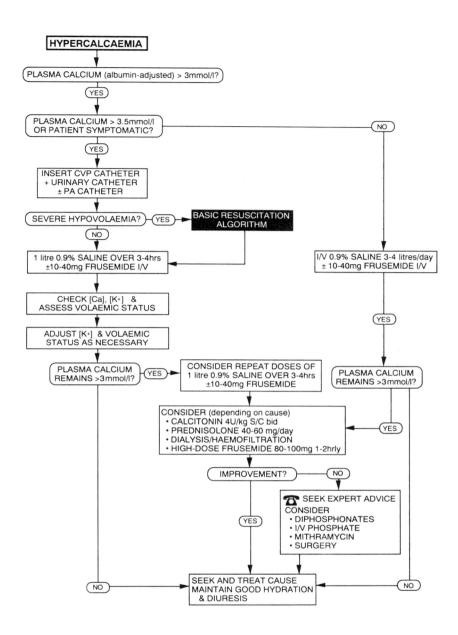

HYPERCALCAEMIA

PLASMA CALCIUM (albumin-adjusted) > 3mmol/l?
— YES

PLASMA CALCIUM > 3.5mmol/l
OR PATIENT SYMPTOMATIC? ——————————————— NO
— YES

INSERT CVP CATHETER
+ URINARY CATHETER
± PA CATHETER

SEVERE HYPOVOLAEMIA? — YES → **BASIC RESUSCITATION ALGORITHM**
— NO

1 litre 0.9% SALINE OVER 3-4hrs
±10-40mg FRUSEMIDE I/V

I/V 0.9% SALINE 3-4 litres/day
± 10-40mg FRUSEMIDE I/V

CHECK [Ca], [K+] &
ASSESS VOLAEMIC STATUS

ADJUST [K+] & VOLAEMIC
STATUS AS NECESSARY

PLASMA CALCIUM
REMAINS >3mmol/l? — YES → CONSIDER REPEAT DOSES OF
1 litre 0.9% SALINE OVER 3-4hrs
±10-40mg FRUSEMIDE

— YES

PLASMA CALCIUM
REMAINS >3mmol/l?

CONSIDER (depending on cause)
• CALCITONIN 4U/kg S/C bid
• PREDNISOLONE 40-60 mg/day
• DIALYSIS/HAEMOFILTRATION
• HIGH-DOSE FRUSEMIDE 80-100mg 1-2hrly

— YES

IMPROVEMENT? —— NO

☎ SEEK EXPERT ADVICE
CONSIDER
• DIPHOSPHONATES
• I/V PHOSPHATE
• MITHRAMYCIN
• SURGERY

— YES

NO → SEEK AND TREAT CAUSE
MAINTAIN GOOD HYDRATION
& DIURESIS ← NO

5.6 Hypocalcaemia

1. Symptoms include tetany (including carpopedal spasm), perioral parasthesiae, hypotension.
2. A prolonged QT interval is seen on the ECG.
3. Chvostek and Trousseau's signs are good clinical indicators of hypocalcaemia.

Causes

1. Associated with hyperphosphataemia:
   - chronic renal failure
   - hypoparathyroidism (including surgery), pseudohypoparathyroidism
2. Associated with low/normal phosphate:
   - osteomalacia
   - overhydration
   - pancreatitis
3. Hypomagnesaemia (e.g. following diuretics, diarrhoea, starvation) is a frequent cause of hypocalcaemia that fails to correct with therapy.
4. Hyperventilation causes a decreased ionized fraction of calcium through the respiratory alkalosis.

Correction for albumin

A number of formulae exist for correcting calcium to the plasma albumin level e.g. add or subtract 0.1 mmol/l calcium for every 6 g/l albumin below/above 42 g/l respectively.

Bibliography

Kanis JA, Yates AJ. Measuring serum calcium. *BMJ* 1985; **290**: 728
Rizzoli R, Bonjour JP. Management of disorders of calcium homeostasis. *Ballieres Clin Endocrinol Metab* 1992; **6**: 129
Zaloga GP. Hypocalcemia in critically ill patients. *Crit Care Med* 1992; **20**: 251

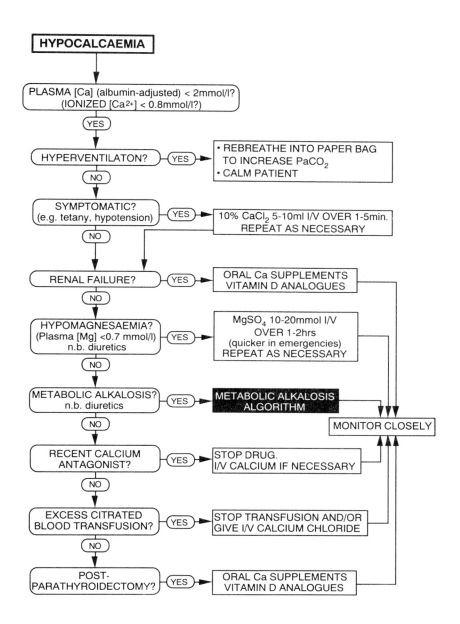

HYPOCALCAEMIA

PLASMA [Ca] (albumin-adjusted) < 2mmol/l?
(IONIZED [Ca^{2+}] < 0.8mmol/l?)

YES

HYPERVENTILATON? — YES →
- REBREATHE INTO PAPER BAG TO INCREASE $PaCO_2$
- CALM PATIENT

NO

SYMPTOMATIC?
(e.g. tetany, hypotension) — YES →
10% $CaCl_2$ 5-10ml I/V OVER 1-5min.
REPEAT AS NECESSARY

NO

RENAL FAILURE? — YES →
ORAL Ca SUPPLEMENTS
VITAMIN D ANALOGUES

NO

HYPOMAGNESAEMIA?
(Plasma [Mg] <0.7 mmol/l)
n.b. diuretics — YES →
$MgSO_4$ 10-20mmol I/V
OVER 1-2hrs
(quicker in emergencies)
REPEAT AS NECESSARY

NO

METABOLIC ALKALOSIS?
n.b. diuretics — YES →
METABOLIC ALKALOSIS
ALGORITHM

NO

MONITOR CLOSELY

RECENT CALCIUM
ANTAGONIST? — YES →
STOP DRUG.
I/V CALCIUM IF NECESSARY

NO

EXCESS CITRATED
BLOOD TRANSFUSION? — YES →
STOP TRANSFUSION AND/OR
GIVE I/V CALCIUM CHLORIDE

NO

POST-
PARATHYROIDECTOMY? — YES →
ORAL Ca SUPPLEMENTS
VITAMIN D ANALOGUES

5.7 Hyperthermia

General
1. Hyperthermia is defined as a core temperature > 41°C
2. Delirium occurs between 40 and 42°C, coma above 42–43°C,
3. The nervous system is most commonly and severely affected.
4. Signs:
   - confusion, delirium, convulsions, pupillary abnormalities, coma
   - tachycardia, ECG changes (ST depression and T wave flattening)
   - later cardiac failure
   - tachypnoea, respiratory alkalosis
   - loss of water, Na^+, K^+, Ca^{++}, Mg^{++} from excessive sweating
   - acute renal failure, rhabdomyolysis
   - thrombocytopenia, DIC, haemolysis

Pyrogen-induced fever
1. Fever is a symptom due to the action of pyrogens on the central nervous system resetting the thermo-regulatory mechanisms.
2. Cooling should usually be aided by antipyretics e.g. aspirin or paracetamol.
3. High fevers with circulatory instability may require active surface cooling.

Heat stroke
1. Body heat production is in excess of ability to dissipate heat
   - high environmental temperature
   - high environmental humidity
   - reduced sweat production (hypovolaemia, anticholinergics)
   - peripheral vasoconstriction (hypovolaemia, cardiac failure)
   - prolonged, vigorous exercise
2. Treatment requires rapid, active cooling.

Malignant hyperthermia
1. Drug-induced myopathy associated with a hereditary calcium transfer defect.
2. Heat production increased by muscle catabolism, muscle spasm and peripheral vasoconstriction.
3. Treatment is based on stopping the offending drug, active cooling, dantrolene 1 mg/kg I/V every 5 min to a maximum dose of 10 mg, mechanical ventilation with high FiO_2, and correction of hyperkalaemia.

Neuroleptic malignant syndrome
1. Hyperthermia is associated with muscle rigidity, akinesia, impaired consciousness and autonomic dysfunction. Recovery takes 1–2 weeks.
2. Treatment is based on stopping the offending agent, active cooling, dopamine agonists (L-dopa + carbidopa, bromocriptine) and dantrolene.

Active cooling
1. Rapid cooling should be instituted for core temperatures >41°C.
2. Remove clothing and use ice packs. Consider cool (iced) bath.
3. Consider bladder, gastric and peritoneal lavage with iced saline.
4. Wet skin, warm and circulate surrounding air to increase evaporative losses.
5. Consider phenothiazines (paralysis if ventilated) to stop shivering.
6. Minimize handling.
7. Stop active cooling when core temp <39°C.

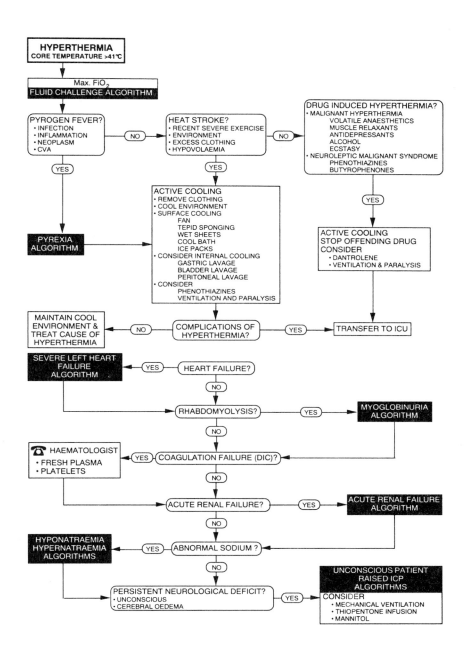

HYPERTHERMIA
CORE TEMPERATURE >41℃

Max. FiO₂
FLUID CHALLENGE ALGORITHM

PYROGEN FEVER?
• INFECTION
• INFLAMMATION
• NEOPLASM
• CVA

— NO —

HEAT STROKE?
• RECENT SEVERE EXERCISE
• ENVIRONMENT
• EXCESS CLOTHING
• HYPOVOLAEMIA

— NO —

DRUG INDUCED HYPERTHERMIA?
• MALIGNANT HYPERTHERMIA
    VOLATILE ANAESTHETICS
    MUSCLE RELAXANTS
    ANTIDEPRESSANTS
    ALCOHOL
    ECSTASY
• NEUROLEPTIC MALIGNANT SYNDROME
    PHENOTHIAZINES
    BUTYROPHENONES

YES

YES

YES

ACTIVE COOLING
• REMOVE CLOTHING
• COOL ENVIRONMENT
• SURFACE COOLING
    FAN
    TEPID SPONGING
    WET SHEETS
    COOL BATH
    ICE PACKS
• CONSIDER INTERNAL COOLING
    GASTRIC LAVAGE
    BLADDER LAVAGE
    PERITONEAL LAVAGE
• CONSIDER
    PHENOTHIAZINES
    VENTILATION AND PARALYSIS

ACTIVE COOLING
STOP OFFENDING DRUG
CONSIDER
    • DANTROLENE
    • VENTILATION & PARALYSIS

PYREXIA
ALGORITHM

MAINTAIN COOL
ENVIRONMENT &
TREAT CAUSE OF
HYPERTHERMIA

— NO —

COMPLICATIONS OF
HYPERTHERMIA?

— YES —

TRANSFER TO ICU

SEVERE LEFT HEART
FAILURE
ALGORITHM

— YES —

HEART FAILURE?

NO

RHABDOMYOLYSIS?

— YES —

MYOGLOBINURIA
ALGORITHM

NO

☎ HAEMATOLOGIST
• FRESH PLASMA
• PLATELETS

— YES —

COAGULATION FAILURE (DIC)?

NO

ACUTE RENAL FAILURE?

— YES —

ACUTE RENAL FAILURE
ALGORITHM

NO

HYPONATRAEMIA
HYPERNATRAEMIA
ALGORITHMS

— YES —

ABNORMAL SODIUM ?

NO

PERSISTENT NEUROLOGICAL DEFICIT?
• UNCONSCIOUS
• CEREBRAL OEDEMA

— YES —

UNCONSCIOUS PATIENT
RAISED ICP
ALGORITHMS
CONSIDER
    • MECHANICAL VENTILATION
    • THIOPENTONE INFUSION
    • MANNITOL

Bibliography

Aun C. Thermal syndromes. In: Oh TE (Ed.) Intensive care manual. 3rd edition. Butterworths, Sydney, 1990, pp 470

Bernheim HA, Block LH, Atkins E. Fever: pathogenesis, pathophysiology and purpose. *Ann Intern Med* 1979; **91**:261

Harchelroad F. Acute thermoregulatory disorders. *Clin Geriatr Med* 1993; **9**:621

Heiman PT. Neuroleptic malignant syndrome and malignant hyperthermia. Important issues for the medical consultant. *Med Clin North Am* 1993; **77**:477

Simon HB. Hyperthermia. *N Engl J Med* 1993; **329**:483

Stitt JT. Fever versus hyperthermia. *Fed Proc* 1979; **38**:39

Notes

5.8 Hypothermia

Clinical features

1. Clinical features and prognosis depend on the degree and duration of hypothermia.
2. Above 33°C shivering usually predominates in an attempt to correct hypothermia.
3. Neurological signs of dysarthria and slowness may appear below 33°C.
4. Below 31°C muscles become hypertonic with sluggish reflexes. Neurological and cardiovascular dysfunction become life threatening.
5. Heart rate and respiratory rate fall with decreasing temperature; blood pressure is reduced below 30°C, arterial pulses often becoming impalpable below 28°C.
6. ECG changes include sinus bradycardia followed by atrial flutter or fibrillation with ventricular ectopics. Thereafter atrial activity may cease. The PR interval, QRS complex and QT interval are prolonged with ST segment depression. The J wave is most frequently seen below 31°C.
7. Ventricular fibrillation is common below 30°C giving way to asystole below 28°C. Hypothermic cardiac arrest associated with rigidity is difficult to distinguish from death.

Rewarming

1. All hypothermic patients with no evidence of other fatal disease should be assumed fully recoverable.
2. Spontaneous rewarming rate is inversely proportional to the duration of hypothermia.
3. Passive spontaneous rewarming with good insulation can achieve a rewarming rate of 0.1–0.7°C/hr.
4. Core temperature may fall during rewarming as cold blood from the periphery is returned to the central circulation.
5. Active surface rewarming can achieve rewarming rates of 1–7°C/hr. Haemodynamic changes may be dramatic so active techniques must be used with caution or avoided in those with cardiovascular disease.
6. Rapid central rewarming with peritoneal dialysis or gastric lavage can achieve rewarming rates of 1–1.5°C/hr; extracorporeal rewarming achieves rates of 3–15°C/hr. The advantages of these techniques include rapid rewarming of the heart during cardiac arrest.

Complications of hypothermia

1. Hypoxaemia is common due to hypoventilation and ventilation perfusion mismatch. Arterial PO_2 corrected for hypothermia is low but often adequate for reduced metabolic demands. Correction of hypoxaemia is more important during rewarming.
2. Hypocapnia should be avoided during mechanical ventilation for hypothermia since the increased affinity of haemoglobin for oxygen is further compounded.
3. Hypovolaemia is common during hypothermia and becomes more severe during rewarming.
4. Metabolic acidosis is common and may be due to reduced tissue oxygen supply, reduced hepatic function and reduced renal function. During rewarming metabolic acidosis may be increased due to shivering and acid washout from reperfused tissues.
5. Initially hypothermia is associated with a diuresis but renal tubular damage follows as renal blood flow is reduced.
6. Acute pancreatitis and acute gastric erosions are not infrequent complications of hypothermia.

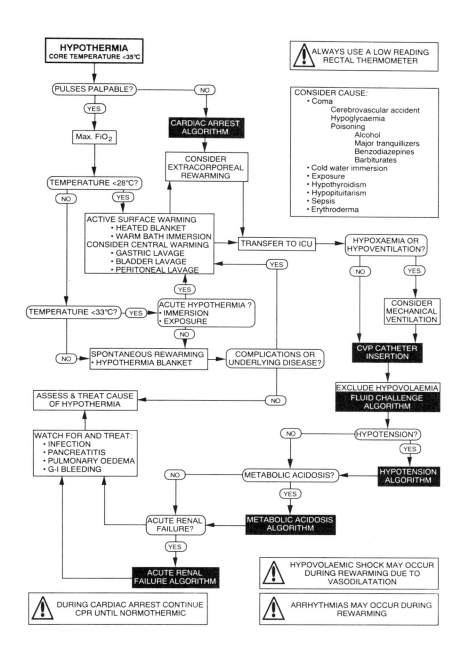

HYPOTHERMIA
CORE TEMPERATURE <35℃

PULSES PALPABLE? — NO

YES

Max. FiO₂

TEMPERATURE <28°C?

NO   YES

CARDIAC ARREST
ALGORITHM

CONSIDER
EXTRACORPOREAL
REWARMING

ALWAYS USE A LOW READING
RECTAL THERMOMETER

CONSIDER CAUSE:
• Coma
    Cerebrovascular accident
    Hypoglycaemia
    Poisoning
        Alcohol
        Major tranquillizers
        Benzodiazepines
        Barbiturates
• Cold water immersion
• Exposure
• Hypothyroidism
• Hypopituitarism
• Sepsis
• Erythroderma

ACTIVE SURFACE WARMING
• HEATED BLANKET
• WARM BATH IMMERSION
CONSIDER CENTRAL WARMING
• GASTRIC LAVAGE
• BLADDER LAVAGE
• PERITONEAL LAVAGE

TRANSFER TO ICU

HYPOXAEMIA OR
HYPOVENTILATION?

YES

NO   YES

ACUTE HYPOTHERMIA ?
• IMMERSION
• EXPOSURE

YES

CONSIDER
MECHANICAL
VENTILATION

TEMPERATURE <33°C? — YES

NO

YES

NO

SPONTANEOUS REWARMING
• HYPOTHERMIA BLANKET

COMPLICATIONS OR
UNDERLYING DISEASE?

CVP CATHETER
INSERTION

EXCLUDE HYPOVOLAEMIA
FLUID CHALLENGE
ALGORITHM

ASSESS & TREAT CAUSE
OF HYPOTHERMIA

NO

WATCH FOR AND TREAT:
• INFECTION
• PANCREATITIS
• PULMONARY OEDEMA
• G-I BLEEDING

NO   HYPOTENSION?

YES

NO   METABOLIC ACIDOSIS?

HYPOTENSION
ALGORITHM

YES

ACUTE RENAL
FAILURE?

METABOLIC ACIDOSIS
ALGORITHM

YES

ACUTE RENAL
FAILURE ALGORITHM

HYPOVOLAEMIC SHOCK MAY OCCUR
DURING REWARMING DUE TO
VASODILATATION

DURING CARDIAC ARREST CONTINUE
CPR UNTIL NORMOTHERMIC

ARRHYTHMIAS MAY OCCUR DURING
REWARMING

Bibliography

Gooden BA. Why some people do not drown. Hypothermia versus the diving response. *Med J Aust* 1992; **157**:629

Harari A, Regnier B, Rapin M, *et al.* Haemodynamic study of prolonged deep accidental hypothermia. *Intensive Care Med* 1975; **1**:65

Harchelroad F. Acute thermoregulatory disorders. *Clin Geriatr Med* 1993; **9**:621

Jolly BT, Ghezzi KT. Accidental hypothermia. *Emerg Med Clin North Am* 1992; **10**:311

Letsou GV, Kopf GS, Elefteriades JA, *et al.* Is cardiopulmonary bypass effective for treatment of hypothermic arrest due to drowning or exposure. *Arch Surg* 1992; **127**:525

MacLean D, Emslie-Smith D. Accidental hypothermia. Blackwell Scientific Publications, Oxford, 1977

Read AE, Emslie-Smith D, Gough KR, *et al.* Pancreatitis and accidental hypothermia. *Lancet* 1961; **ii**:1219

Reuler JB. Hypothermia: pathophysiology, clinical settings and management. *Ann Intern Med* 1978; **89**:519

Rosenfield JB. Acid-base and electrolyte disturbances in hypothermia. *Am J Cardiol* 1963; **12**:678

Weinberg AD. Hypothermia. *Ann Emerg Med* 1993; **22**:370

Notes

5.9 Metabolic acidosis

Treatment should always be directed at the underlying cause rather than manipulation of the pH.

Sodium bicarbonate therapy

1. The $PaCO_2$ may rise if minute volume is not increased. This may result in intracellular acidosis which can depress myocardial cell function.
2. The decrease in plasma ionized calcium may also cause a decrease in myocardial contractility. Significantly worse haemodynamic effects have been reported with bicarbonate compared to equimolar saline in patients with severe heart failure.
3. There is no human evidence that bicarbonate improves myocardial contractility or increases the response to circulating catecholamines in acidosis. Haemodynamic responses to sodium bicarbonate and equimolar sodium chloride solutions were shown to be similar in ICU patients with lactic acidosis; the hypertonicity of the bicarbonate solution appears more significant than its alkalinizing effect. The acidosis relating to myocardial depression is related to intracellular changes which are not accurately reflected by arterial blood chemistry.
4. Bicarbonate may cause hyperosmolality, hypernatraemia, hypokalaemia and sodium overload.
5. Bicarbonate may cause arterial hypoxaemia and decreased tissue oxygenation.
6. Sodium bicarbonate does have a place in the management of acid retention or alkali loss, e.g. chronic renal failure, renal tubular acidosis, fistulae, etc. Replacement of fluid and potassium losses should be attempted first.

Miscellaneous

1. Though offering theoretical advantages, buffers such as Carbicarb and THAM (tri-hydroxy-methyl-aminomethane) have not been demonstrated to be superior to bicarbonate in the treatment of acidotic adults.
2. Type B lactic acidosis, i.e. lactaemia in the presence of adequate organ perfusion, may occur from a number of rare causes, e.g. phenformin therapy, fructose infusion, sorbitol, ethylene glycol. Aim treatment at discontinuing the causative factor and, possibly, using bicarbonate if the patient is very symptomatic.

Bibliography

Arieff AI. Treatment of metabolic acidosis in low flow states: should we administer bicarbonate? In: Vincent JL, (Ed.) Update in intensive care and emergency medicine No.8. Springer-Verlag, Berlin. 1989, p 322

Arieff AI. Indications for use of bicarbonate in patients with metabolic acidosis. *Br J Anaesth* 1991; **67**:165

Bersin RM, Arieff AI. Improved hemodynamic function during hypoxia with carbicarb, a new buffering agent for the management of acidosis. *Circulation* 1988; **77**:227

Bersin RM, Chatterjee K, Arieff AI. Metabolic and hemodynamic consequences of sodium bicarbonate administration in patients with heart disease. *Am J Med* 1989; **87**:5

Cooper DJ, Walley KR, Wiggs BR, Russell JA. Bicarbonate does not improve hemodynamics in critically ill patients who have lactic acidosis. *Ann Intern Med* 1990; **112**:492

Graf H, Leach W, Arieff AI. Evidence for a detrimental effect of bicarbonate therapy in hypoxic lactic acidosis. *Science* 1985; **227**:754

Makisalo HJ, Soini HO, Nordin AJ, Hockerstedt KAV. Effects of bicarbonate therapy on tissue oxygenation during resuscitation of hemorrhagic shock. *Crit Care Med* 1989; **17**: 1170

Narins RG, Cohen JJ. Bicarbonate therapy for organic acidosis: The case for its continued use. *Ann Intern Med* 1987; **106**:615

Stacpoole PW. Lactic acidosis:the case against bicarbonate therapy. *Ann Intern Med* 1986; **105**:276

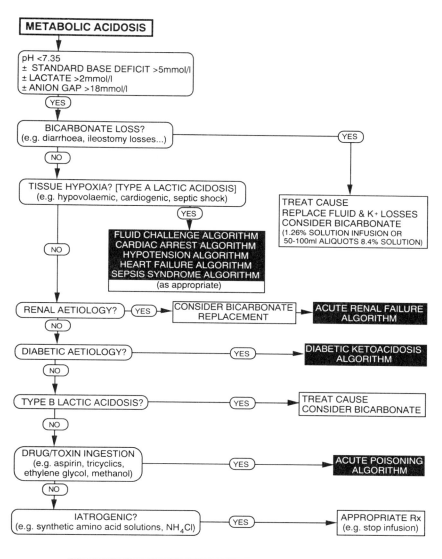

METABOLIC ACIDOSIS

pH <7.35
± STANDARD BASE DEFICIT >5mmol/l
± LACTATE >2mmol/l
± ANION GAP >18mmol/l

(YES)

BICARBONATE LOSS? ─────────────────────── (YES)
(e.g. diarrhoea, ileostomy losses...)

(NO)

TISSUE HYPOXIA? [TYPE A LACTIC ACIDOSIS]
(e.g. hypovolaemic, cardiogenic, septic shock)

(YES)

TREAT CAUSE
REPLACE FLUID & K+ LOSSES
CONSIDER BICARBONATE
(1.26% SOLUTION INFUSION OR
50-100ml ALIQUOTS 8.4% SOLUTION)

FLUID CHALLENGE ALGORITHM
CARDIAC ARREST ALGORITHM
HYPOTENSION ALGORITHM
HEART FAILURE ALGORITHM
SEPSIS SYNDROME ALGORITHM
(as appropriate)

(NO)

RENAL AETIOLOGY? ─(YES)→ CONSIDER BICARBONATE REPLACEMENT ─→ ACUTE RENAL FAILURE ALGORITHM

(NO)

DIABETIC AETIOLOGY? ──────── (YES) ─→ DIABETIC KETOACIDOSIS ALGORITHM

(NO)

TYPE B LACTIC ACIDOSIS? ──────── (YES) ─→ TREAT CAUSE CONSIDER BICARBONATE

(NO)

DRUG/TOXIN INGESTION
(e.g. aspirin, tricyclics,
ethylene glycol, methanol) ──────── (YES) ─→ ACUTE POISONING ALGORITHM

(NO)

IATROGENIC?
(e.g. synthetic amino acid solutions, NH_4Cl) ──── (YES) ─→ APPROPRIATE Rx
(e.g. stop infusion)

⚠ CONSIDER BICARBONATE (1mmol/kg) IF:-
• CAUSE IS NOT ORGAN HYPOPERFUSION
• NO ANURIA,OLIGURIA or FLUID OVERLOAD
• PROLONGED CARDIAC ARREST

5.10 Metabolic alkalosis

Treatment
1. Replacement of fluid, sodium, chloride and potassium losses is often sufficient to restore acid-base balance.
2. Active treatment is rarely necessary. If so, give ammonium chloride 5 g P/O tid.
3. Compensatory metabolic alkalosis for long-standing respiratory acidosis, followed by correction of the acidosis, for instance by mechanical ventilation, will lead to an uncompensated metabolic alkalosis. This will usually correct with time though treatments such as acetazolamide can be considered. Mechanical 'hypoventilation', i.e. maintaining hypercapnia, can also be considered.

Miscellaneous
1. Urinary pH is often acidic in the presence of a significant metabolic alkalosis.
2. Alkalosis is associated with an increased alveolar–arterial oxygen difference and hypoxaemia.
3. Correction of alkalosis causes an increased PaO_2 related to the Bohr effect and to enhanced hypoxic pulmonary vasoconstriction. An unwanted, though possibly transient, effect may be increased pulmonary vascular pressures.

Bibliography
Brimioulle S, Vincent J-L, Dufaye P, Berre J, Degaute JP, Kahn RJ. Hydrochloric acid infusion for treatment of metabolic alkalosis effects on acid-base balance and oxygenation. *Crit Care Med* 1985; **13**: 738
Brimioulle S, Kahn RJ. Effects of metabolic alkalosis on pulmonary gas exchange. *Am Rev Respir Dis* 1990; **141**:1185
Worthley LIG. Acid-base balance and disorders. In: Oh TE (Ed.) *Intensive care manual.* Butterworths, Sydney, 1990, p500

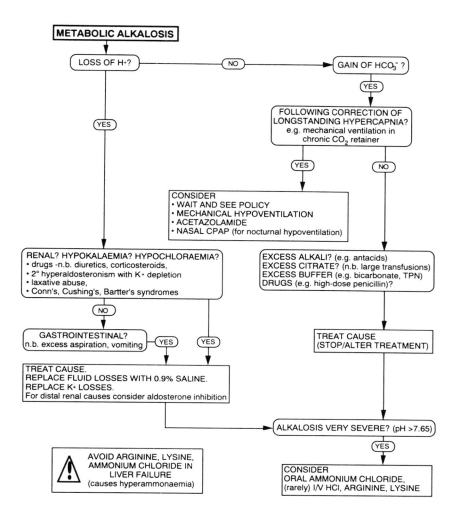

METABOLIC ALKALOSIS

LOSS OF H+? ──NO──→ GAIN OF HCO₃⁻ ?
↓ YES

GAIN OF HCO₃⁻ ? → YES

FOLLOWING CORRECTION OF
LONGSTANDING HYPERCAPNIA?
e.g. mechanical ventilation in
chronic CO₂ retainer

YES / NO

CONSIDER
• WAIT AND SEE POLICY
• MECHANICAL HYPOVENTILATION
• ACETAZOLAMIDE
• NASAL CPAP (for nocturnal hypoventilation)

RENAL? HYPOKALAEMIA? HYPOCHLORAEMIA?
• drugs -n.b. diuretics, corticosteroids,
• 2° hyperaldosteronism with K+ depletion
• laxative abuse,
• Conn's, Cushing's, Bartter's syndromes

NO

EXCESS ALKALI? (e.g. antacids)
EXCESS CITRATE? (n.b. large transfusions)
EXCESS BUFFER (e.g. bicarbonate, TPN)
DRUGS (e.g. high-dose penicillin)?

GASTROINTESTINAL?
n.b. excess aspiration, vomiting — YES / YES

TREAT CAUSE
(STOP/ALTER TREATMENT)

TREAT CAUSE.
REPLACE FLUID LOSSES WITH 0.9% SALINE.
REPLACE K+ LOSSES.
For distal renal causes consider aldosterone inhibition

ALKALOSIS VERY SEVERE? (pH >7.65)

YES

⚠ AVOID ARGININE, LYSINE,
AMMONIUM CHLORIDE IN
LIVER FAILURE
(causes hyperammonaemia)

CONSIDER
ORAL AMMONIUM CHLORIDE,
(rarely) I/V HCl, ARGININE, LYSINE

6. Endocrine

6.1/6.2 Hyperglycaemic emergencies

Fluid and electrolyte management
1. In severe diabetic ketoacidosis (DKA) approximate losses are:
   * water 5–10 litres
   * sodium 400–700 mmol
   * potassium 250–700 mmol
2. The fluid loss is relatively hypotonic (urine sodium concentration is about 55 mmol/l) as about half is derived from the intracellular compartment.
3. Fluid and electrolyte repletion should not follow a strict regimen but must be tailored to individual needs.
4. Fluid replacement with 0.9% saline can be used though caution should be exercised to prevent sodium overload. 5% glucose should be substituted after replacing the sodium debt.
5. Hypotonic (0.45%) saline resuscitation may be appropriate in the non-shocked patient but in shock it is important to restore the circulating blood volume as quickly as possible with colloid solutions.
6. Over-rapid rehydration may result in cerebral oedema. Patients with impaired cardiac or renal function may also be compromised.
7. Infusing insulin causes a large and rapid intracellular shift of potassium leading to hypokalaemia. Early and vigorous potassium replacement is usually needed with frequent monitoring of the plasma level.

Management of hyperglycaemia
1. Hyperglycaemia should be corrected gradually at a rate of 2–4 mmol/hr.
2. The insulin infusion should be continued, even after achieving normoglycaemia, until heavy ketonuria has disappeared and plasma bicarbonate has normalized. Additional glucose (by infusion if necessary) may be required to maintain normoglycaemia.
   n.b. 5% glucose only contains 20 Cal/100 ml.

Other aspects
1. A nasogastric tube should be inserted if the conscious level is impaired as gastric emptying is often delayed and acute gastric dilatation is common; the risk of aspiration is increased.
2. Bicarbonate should not be used routinely, even for severe acidosis. It causes:
   * increased intracellular acidosis
   * depressed respiration due to relative CSF alkalosis
3. Approximately 50% of all cases are related to underlying disease such as sepsis, MI, stroke, infective gastroenteritis.
4. Antibiotics should only be given for proved infection or where there is a high index of clinical suspicion.
5. Abdominal pain should not be dismissed as part of the syndrome.
6. Plasma amylase commonly exceeds 1000 U/l but does not necessarily indicate pancreatitis.
7. The plasma sodium level will often rise with treatment due to a shift of water into the cells and a shift of sodium from the cells in exchange for potassium.
8. Coma need not be present for the condition to be life-threatening.

Hyperosmolar hyperglycaemic non-ketotic states

1. More common in elderly, non-insulin dependent diabetics.
2. Fluid depletion is greater, coma more frequent and mortality much higher than in DKA.
3. Hyperosmolality may predispose to thrombotic events. Unless otherwise contraindicated, these patients should be fully heparinized until full recovery (which may take 5+ days).
4. Hypotonic saline resuscitation should be slow (over 48–72 hrs).
5. Patients may be hypersensitive to insulin and require lower doses. They usually go home on tablets or even diet alone.

Bibliography

Alberti KGMM, Hockaday TDR. Diabetes mellitus. In: Weatherall DJ, Ledingham JG, Warrell DA (Eds.) Oxford Textbook of medicine. Oxford University Press, 1987, 9.51

Arieff AI, Kleeman CR. Studies on mechanisms of cerebral edema in diabetic comas: effects of hyperglycaemia and rapid lowering of plasma glucose in normal rabbits. *J Clin Invest* 1973; **52**:571

Hillman K. Fluid resuscitation in diabetic emergencies—a reappraisal. *Intensive Care Med* 1987; **13**:4

Hillman K. The management of acute diabetic emergencies. *Clinical Intensive Care* 1991; **2**: 154

Richardson JE, Donaldson MDC. Diabetic emergencies. *Prescribers Journal* 1989; **29**:174

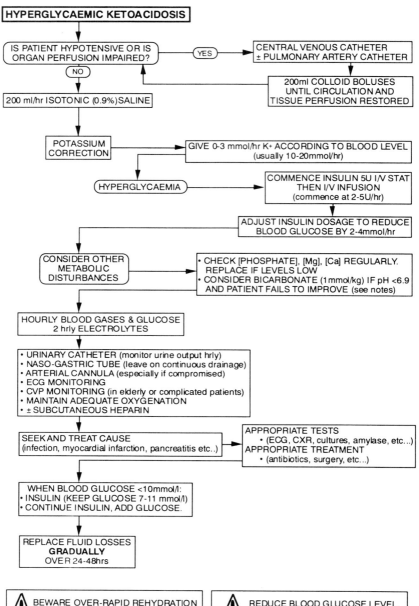

HYPERGLYCAEMIC KETOACIDOSIS

IS PATIENT HYPOTENSIVE OR IS ORGAN PERFUSION IMPAIRED? — YES → CENTRAL VENOUS CATHETER ± PULMONARY ARTERY CATHETER

NO

200ml COLLOID BOLUSES UNTIL CIRCULATION AND TISSUE PERFUSION RESTORED

200 ml/hr ISOTONIC (0.9%) SALINE

POTASSIUM CORRECTION → GIVE 0-3 mmol/hr K+ ACCORDING TO BLOOD LEVEL (usually 10-20mmol/hr)

HYPERGLYCAEMIA → COMMENCE INSULIN 5U I/V STAT THEN I/V INFUSION (commence at 2-5U/hr)

ADJUST INSULIN DOSAGE TO REDUCE BLOOD GLUCOSE BY 2-4mmol/hr

CONSIDER OTHER METABOLIC DISTURBANCES →
• CHECK [PHOSPHATE], [Mg], [Ca] REGULARLY. REPLACE IF LEVELS LOW
• CONSIDER BICARBONATE (1mmol/kg) IF pH <6.9 AND PATIENT FAILS TO IMPROVE (see notes)

HOURLY BLOOD GASES & GLUCOSE 2 hrly ELECTROLYTES

• URINARY CATHETER (monitor urine output hrly)
• NASO-GASTRIC TUBE (leave on continuous drainage)
• ARTERIAL CANNULA (especially if compromised)
• ECG MONITORING
• CVP MONITORING (in elderly or complicated patients)
• MAINTAIN ADEQUATE OXYGENATION
• ± SUBCUTANEOUS HEPARIN

SEEK AND TREAT CAUSE (infection, myocardial infarction, pancreatitis etc..) →
APPROPRIATE TESTS
• (ECG, CXR, cultures, amylase, etc...)
APPROPRIATE TREATMENT
• (antibiotics, surgery, etc...)

WHEN BLOOD GLUCOSE <10mmol/l:
• INSULIN (KEEP GLUCOSE 7-11 mmol/l)
• CONTINUE INSULIN, ADD GLUCOSE.

REPLACE FLUID LOSSES **GRADUALLY** OVER 24-48hrs

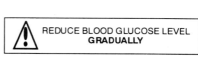

⚠ BEWARE OVER-RAPID REHYDRATION (n.b. heart disease, elderly)

⚠ REDUCE BLOOD GLUCOSE LEVEL **GRADUALLY**

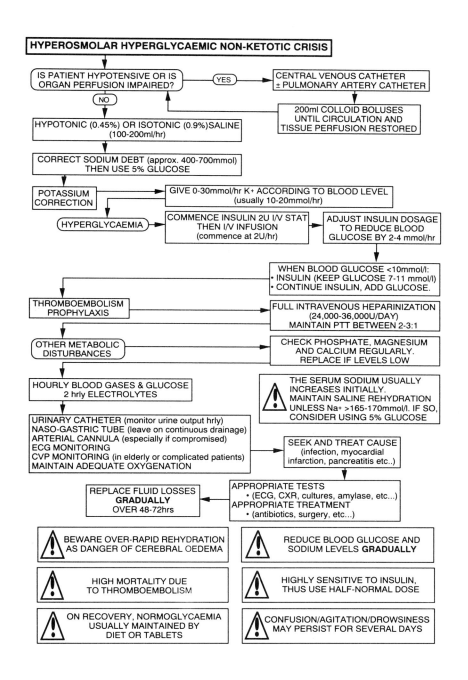

HYPEROSMOLAR HYPERGLYCAEMIC NON-KETOTIC CRISIS

IS PATIENT HYPOTENSIVE OR IS ORGAN PERFUSION IMPAIRED? — (YES) → CENTRAL VENOUS CATHETER ± PULMONARY ARTERY CATHETER

(NO)

200ml COLLOID BOLUSES UNTIL CIRCULATION AND TISSUE PERFUSION RESTORED

HYPOTONIC (0.45%) OR ISOTONIC (0.9%) SALINE (100-200ml/hr)

CORRECT SODIUM DEBT (approx. 400-700mmol) THEN USE 5% GLUCOSE

POTASSIUM CORRECTION → GIVE 0-30mmol/hr K+ ACCORDING TO BLOOD LEVEL (usually 10-20mmol/hr)

(HYPERGLYCAEMIA) → COMMENCE INSULIN 2U I/V STAT THEN I/V INFUSION (commence at 2U/hr) → ADJUST INSULIN DOSAGE TO REDUCE BLOOD GLUCOSE BY 2-4 mmol/hr

WHEN BLOOD GLUCOSE <10mmol/l:
• INSULIN (KEEP GLUCOSE 7-11 mmol/l)
• CONTINUE INSULIN, ADD GLUCOSE.

THROMBOEMBOLISM PROPHYLAXIS → FULL INTRAVENOUS HEPARINIZATION (24,000-36,000U/DAY) MAINTAIN PTT BETWEEN 2-3:1

OTHER METABOLIC DISTURBANCES → CHECK PHOSPHATE, MAGNESIUM AND CALCIUM REGULARLY. REPLACE IF LEVELS LOW

HOURLY BLOOD GASES & GLUCOSE 2 hrly ELECTROLYTES

⚠ THE SERUM SODIUM USUALLY INCREASES INITIALLY. MAINTAIN SALINE REHYDRATION UNLESS Na+ >165-170mmol/l. IF SO, CONSIDER USING 5% GLUCOSE

URINARY CATHETER (monitor urine output hrly)
NASO-GASTRIC TUBE (leave on continuous drainage)
ARTERIAL CANNULA (especially if compromised)
ECG MONITORING
CVP MONITORING (in elderly or complicated patients)
MAINTAIN ADEQUATE OXYGENATION

SEEK AND TREAT CAUSE (infection, myocardial infarction, pancreatitis etc..)

REPLACE FLUID LOSSES **GRADUALLY** OVER 48-72hrs ← APPROPRIATE TESTS
• (ECG, CXR, cultures, amylase, etc...)
APPROPRIATE TREATMENT
• (antibiotics, surgery, etc...)

⚠ BEWARE OVER-RAPID REHYDRATION AS DANGER OF CEREBRAL OEDEMA

⚠ REDUCE BLOOD GLUCOSE AND SODIUM LEVELS **GRADUALLY**

⚠ HIGH MORTALITY DUE TO THROMBOEMBOLISM

⚠ HIGHLY SENSITIVE TO INSULIN, THUS USE HALF-NORMAL DOSE

⚠ ON RECOVERY, NORMOGLYCAEMIA USUALLY MAINTAINED BY DIET OR TABLETS

⚠ CONFUSION/AGITATION/DROWSINESS MAY PERSIST FOR SEVERAL DAYS

6.3 Hypoglycaemia

1. Symptoms include sweating, tachycardia, nausea, vomiting, altered behaviour and conscious level, seizures, acute neurological focal signs.
2. Confused, aggressive behaviour in an inebriated patient may be due to hypoglycaemia.
3. Causes:
   - excess insulin, sulphonylureas
   - malnutrition, starvation
   - alcohol
   - liver failure
   - quinine, aspirin
   - sepsis
   - hypoadrenalism, hypopituitarism, insulinoma
   - post-prandial after gastric surgery
4. Biguanides do not cause hypoglycaemia.
5. 5% glucose solution only contains 20 Cal/100 ml.
6. Long-acting sulphonyl ureas/insulin may have prolonged effects.
7. Quinine therapy for malaria may cause hypoglycaemia.

Bibliography

Alberti KGMM, Hockaday TDR. Diabetes mellitus. In: Weatherall DJ, Ledingham JG, Warrell DA, (Eds.) Oxford Textbook of Medicine. Oxford University Press, 1987, 9.51
Hillman K. The management of acute diabetic emergencies. *Clinical Intensive Care* 1991; **2**:154
Richardson JE, Donaldson MDC. Diabetic emergencies. *Prescribers Journal* 1989; **29**:174

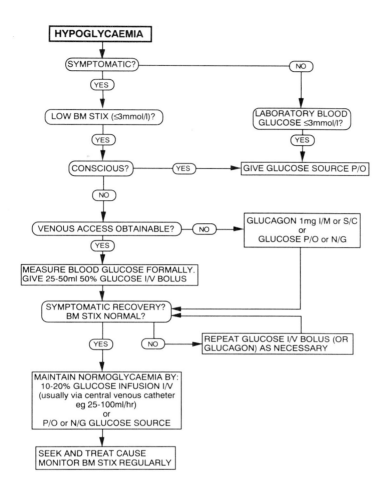

HYPOGLYCAEMIA

SYMPTOMATIC? ──────────────── NO
│   │
YES   ↓
│   LABORATORY BLOOD
↓   GLUCOSE ≤3mmol/l?
LOW BM STIX (≤3mmol/l)?   │
│   YES
YES   │
│   ↓
↓
CONSCIOUS? ── YES ──────────→ GIVE GLUCOSE SOURCE P/O
│
NO
│
↓
VENOUS ACCESS OBTAINABLE? ── NO ──→ GLUCAGON 1mg I/M or S/C
│   or
YES   GLUCOSE P/O or N/G
│
↓
MEASURE BLOOD GLUCOSE FORMALLY.
GIVE 25-50ml 50% GLUCOSE I/V BOLUS
│
↓
SYMPTOMATIC RECOVERY? ←─────────────
BM STIX NORMAL?
│   │
YES   NO ──→ REPEAT GLUCOSE I/V BOLUS (OR
│   GLUCAGON) AS NECESSARY
↓
MAINTAIN NORMOGLYCAEMIA BY:
10-20% GLUCOSE INFUSION I/V
(usually via central venous catheter
eg 25-100ml/hr)
or
P/O or N/G GLUCOSE SOURCE
│
↓
SEEK AND TREAT CAUSE
MONITOR BM STIX REGULARLY

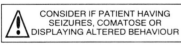

CONSIDER IF PATIENT HAVING SEIZURES, COMATOSE OR DISPLAYING ALTERED BEHAVIOUR

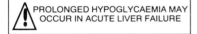

PROLONGED HYPOGLYCAEMIA MAY OCCUR IN ACUTE LIVER FAILURE

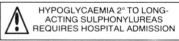

HYPOGLYCAEMIA 2° TO LONG-ACTING SULPHONYLUREAS REQUIRES HOSPITAL ADMISSION

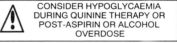

CONSIDER HYPOGLYCAEMIA DURING QUININE THERAPY OR POST-ASPIRIN OR ALCOHOL OVERDOSE

6.4 Thyrotoxic crisis

Clinical features

1. Clinical features are usually an exacerbation of features of hyperthyroidism.
2. Cardiovascular complications may be dominant in older patients.
3. The elderly may have few features of hyperthyroidism, having progressed to a state of lethargy possibly through exhaustion; sudden death is common in these patients.
4. Thyroid hormone levels are no different to those found in severe hyperthyroidism.

Precipitating factors

1. There is usually a concurrent event precipitating the crisis.
2. Thyrotoxic crisis usually occurs in patients with pre-existing hyperthyroidism but may be the presenting feature.
3. It is essential to render patients euthyroid before surgical manipulation of the thyroid gland.
4. ^{131}I therapy for hyperthyroidism may precipitate thyrotoxic crisis probably via radiation thyroiditis; pretreatment prevents this complication.

Thyroid function tests

1. Raised thyroxine levels may be due to increased circulating thyroid binding proteins, e.g. in pregnancy or oestrogen treatment, with phenothiazine treatment or in viral hepatitis.
2. To ensure that raised serum thyroxine levels are indicative of hyperthyroidism assay of free thyroxine is necessary. Alternatively, an estimate of unoccupied sites on thyroid binding protein can be made with a T3 uptake test to allow calculation of a free thyroxine index.
3. TSH levels will be low in primary hyperthyroidism.

Treatment

1. Treatment aims to block thyroid hormone synthesis, block release of thyroid hormone and block the effects of circulating thyroid hormones.
2. Treatment should be via the oral or nasogastric route where possible.
3. Severe crisis is acutely life-threatening and should be managed in an intensive care environment.
4. Treatment of the precipitating cause is a major determinant of outcome.

Bibliography

Burch HB, Wartofsky L. Life-threatening thyrotoxicosis. Thyroid storm. *Endocrinol Metab Clin North Am* 1993; **22**:263

Burger AG, Philippe J. Thyroid emergencies. *Baillieres Clin Endocrinol Metab* 1992; **6**:77

Cruetzig H, Kallfelz I, Haindl J. Thyroid storm and iodine 131 treatment. *Lancet* 1976; ii:145

Ikram H. Haemodynamic effects of beta-adrenergic blockade in hyperthyroid patients with and without heart failure. *Br Med J* 1977; **1**:1505

Isley WL. Thyroid dysfunction in the severely ill and elderly. Forget the classic signs and symptoms. *Postgrad Med* 1993; **94**:111

Smallridge RC. Metabolic and anatomic thyroid emergencies: a review. *Crit Care Med* 1992; **20**:276

Woeber KA. Thyrotoxicosis and the heart. *N Engl J Med* 1992; **327**:94

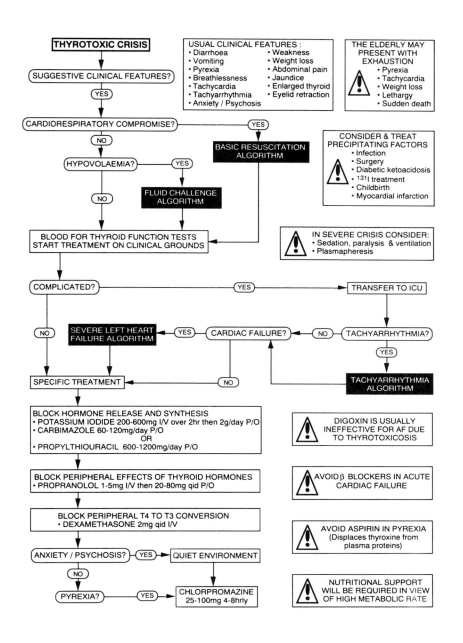

THYROTOXIC CRISIS

SUGGESTIVE CLINICAL FEATURES? — YES

USUAL CLINICAL FEATURES :
- Diarrhoea
- Vomiting
- Pyrexia
- Breathlessness
- Tachycardia
- Tachyarrhythmia
- Anxiety / Psychosis
- Weakness
- Weight loss
- Abdominal pain
- Jaundice
- Enlarged thyroid
- Eyelid retraction

THE ELDERLY MAY PRESENT WITH EXHAUSTION
- Pyrexia
- Tachycardia
- Weight loss
- Lethargy
- Sudden death

CARDIORESPIRATORY COMPROMISE? — YES

NO

BASIC RESUSCITATION ALGORITHM

HYPOVOLAEMIA? — YES

NO

FLUID CHALLENGE ALGORITHM

CONSIDER & TREAT PRECIPITATING FACTORS
- Infection
- Surgery
- Diabetic ketoacidosis
- 131I treatment
- Childbirth
- Myocardial infarction

BLOOD FOR THYROID FUNCTION TESTS
START TREATMENT ON CLINICAL GROUNDS

IN SEVERE CRISIS CONSIDER:
- Sedation, paralysis & ventilation
- Plasmapheresis

COMPLICATED? — YES — TRANSFER TO ICU

NO

SEVERE LEFT HEART FAILURE ALGORITHM — YES — CARDIAC FAILURE? — NO — TACHYARRHYTHMIA?

YES

TACHYARRHYTHMIA ALGORITHM

SPECIFIC TREATMENT — NO

BLOCK HORMONE RELEASE AND SYNTHESIS
- POTASSIUM IODIDE 200-600mg I/V over 2hr then 2g/day P/O
- CARBIMAZOLE 60-120mg/day P/O
OR
- PROPYLTHIOURACIL 600-1200mg/day P/O

DIGOXIN IS USUALLY INEFFECTIVE FOR AF DUE TO THYROTOXICOSIS

BLOCK PERIPHERAL EFFECTS OF THYROID HORMONES
- PROPRANOLOL 1-5mg I/V then 20-80mg qid P/O

AVOID β BLOCKERS IN ACUTE CARDIAC FAILURE

BLOCK PERIPHERAL T4 TO T3 CONVERSION
- DEXAMETHASONE 2mg qid I/V

AVOID ASPIRIN IN PYREXIA
(Displaces thyroxine from plasma proteins)

ANXIETY / PSYCHOSIS? — YES → QUIET ENVIRONMENT

NO

PYREXIA? — YES → CHLORPROMAZINE 25-100mg 4-8hrly

NUTRITIONAL SUPPORT WILL BE REQUIRED IN VIEW OF HIGH METABOLIC RATE

6.5 Myxoedema coma

Clinical features
1. Clinical features are an exacerbation of the features of hypothyroidism.
2. Hypothermia is common but not invariable.
3. Acidosis may be secondary to hypoventilation with CO_2 retention or lactate accumulation due to poor tissue perfusion.
4. Hyponatraemia is usually due to inappropriate ADH secretion.
5. Normochromic, normocytic anaemia is common in hypothyroidism but macrocytic anaemia may be due to co-existent autoimmune pernicious anaemia and microcytic anaemia may be due to menorrhagia.

Thyroid function tests
1. Serum thyroid hormones can be measured by radioimmunoassay.
2. TSH levels will be high in primary hypothyroidism.

Treatment
1. Treatment of complications of severe hypothyroidism is more important than thyroid hormone replacement.
2. Thyroid hormone replacement should be via the oral or nasogastric route where possible.
3. Mortality from myxoedema coma is 50%; most cases should be managed in an intensive care environment.
4. Steroid therapy should be given for co-existing hypoadrenalism, signs of which may be masked by myxoedema:
   • low metabolic rate may prevent the adrenals responding to stress
   • associated autoimmune hypoadrenalism
   • hypothyroidism and hypoadrenalism may be due to hypopituitarism
5. Several regimens for replacing thyroid hormones have been described:
   • T3 replacement starting at low doses
   • T3 replacement starting at full doses
   • high dose T4 replacement
   • combination therapy with T3 and T4
6. High dose replacement regimens are potentially dangerous and offer no real advantages. If the metabolic rate is increased too rapidly there may be cardiovascular decompensation.
7. Starting treatment with T3 offers several potential advantages:
   • effect is more rapid
   • T4 must be converted to T3 for effect
   • half life of T4 is prolonged in hypothyroidism
8. There are several disadvantages of starting treatment with T3:
   • less predictable effect than T4
   • short half life gives peak and trough effect
9. 20 μg T3 is equivalent to 100 μg T4.

Bibliography
Burger AG, Philippe J. Thyroid emergencies. *Baillieres Clin Endocrinol Metab* 1992; **6**:77
Evered D, Hall R. Hypothyroidism. *Br Med J* 1972; **1**:290
Isley WL. Thyroid dysfunction in the severely ill and elderly. Forget the classic signs and symptoms. *Postgrad Med* 1993; **94**:111
Smallridge RC. Metabolic and anatomic thyroid emergencies: a review. *Crit Care Med* 1992; **20**:276
Woods KL, Holmes GK. Myxoedema coma presenting in status epilepticus. *Postgrad Med J* 1977; **53**:46

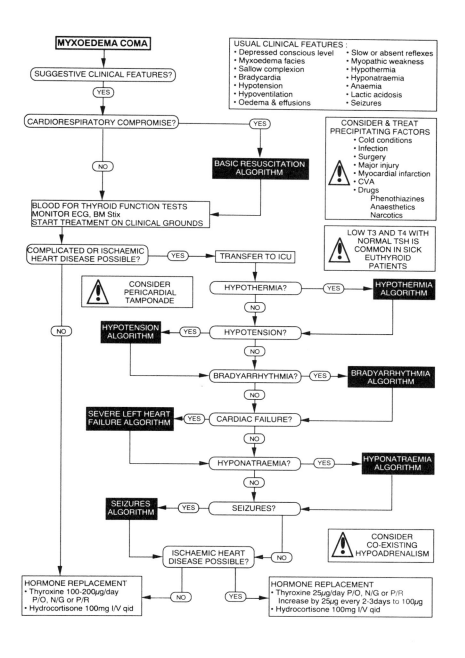

MYXOEDEMA COMA

SUGGESTIVE CLINICAL FEATURES? — YES

USUAL CLINICAL FEATURES :
- Depressed conscious level
- Myxoedema facies
- Sallow complexion
- Bradycardia
- Hypotension
- Hypoventilation
- Oedema & effusions
- Slow or absent reflexes
- Myopathic weakness
- Hypothermia
- Hyponatraemia
- Anaemia
- Lactic acidosis
- Seizures

CARDIORESPIRATORY COMPROMISE? — YES → BASIC RESUSCITATION ALGORITHM

NO

CONSIDER & TREAT PRECIPITATING FACTORS
- Cold conditions
- Infection
- Surgery
- Major injury
- Myocardial infarction
- CVA
- Drugs
  Phenothiazines
  Anaesthetics
  Narcotics

BLOOD FOR THYROID FUNCTION TESTS
MONITOR ECG, BM Stix
START TREATMENT ON CLINICAL GROUNDS

LOW T3 AND T4 WITH NORMAL TSH IS COMMON IN SICK EUTHYROID PATIENTS

COMPLICATED OR ISCHAEMIC HEART DISEASE POSSIBLE? — YES → TRANSFER TO ICU

NO

CONSIDER PERICARDIAL TAMPONADE

HYPOTHERMIA? — YES → HYPOTHERMIA ALGORITHM

NO

HYPOTENSION ALGORITHM ← YES — HYPOTENSION?

NO

BRADYARRHYTHMIA? — YES → BRADYARRHYTHMIA ALGORITHM

NO

SEVERE LEFT HEART FAILURE ALGORITHM ← YES — CARDIAC FAILURE?

NO

HYPONATRAEMIA? — YES → HYPONATRAEMIA ALGORITHM

NO

SEIZURES ALGORITHM ← YES — SEIZURES?

NO

CONSIDER CO-EXISTING HYPOADRENALISM

ISCHAEMIC HEART DISEASE POSSIBLE?

HORMONE REPLACEMENT
- Thyroxine 100-200µg/day P/O, N/G or P/R
- Hydrocortisone 100mg I/V qid

NO ← → YES

HORMONE REPLACEMENT
- Thyroxine 25µg/day P/O, N/G or P/R Increase by 25µg every 2-3days to 100µg
- Hydrocortisone 100mg I/V qid

6.6 Hypoadrenal crisis

Clinical features
1. Dysfunction of adrenal cortex leads to clinical features of both glucocorticoid and mineralocorticoid deficiency.
2. In primary hypoadrenalism pigmentation is due to ACTH excess. Scrotal and axillary pigmentation are more common than buccal pigmentation.
3. Salt depletion and postural hypotension reflect mineralocorticoid deficiency and are therefore commonly absent in patients with hypoadrenalism secondary to hypopituitarism.
4. It is the salt and water loss of mineralocorticoid deficiency that is immediately life-threatening in primary hypoadrenalism.

Treatment and investigation
1. Urgent treatment of salt and water deficiency is life-saving.
2. Glucocorticoid replacement should be with hydrocortisone rather than insoluble steroid acetates such as cortisone or prednisone; these have to be converted to the soluble steroid for effect.
3. The precipitating cause should be diagnosed and treated.
4. Mineralocorticoid replacement is only required after the acute crisis has been corrected and as part of maintenance treatment.
5. Maintenance glucocorticoid therapy usually requires 30 mg hydrocortisone daily given as 20 mg in the morning and 10 mg in the afternoon.
6. The acute phase of treatment should not be delayed by a Synacthen test .
7. Co-existing autoimmune hypothyroidism requires evidence of thyroid antibodies for diagnosis. Low T4 and high TSH may occur with hypoadrenalism and respond to steroid therapy.

Steroid withdrawal hypoadrenalism
1. Prolonged (> 2 weeks) treatment with pharmacological doses of corticosteroids will suppress ACTH secretion from the pituitary.
2. After 8–10 years there will be irreversible adrenal atrophy.
3. Sudden withdrawal of steroid therapy will lead to glucocorticoid deficiency.
4. Failure to increase steroid dose to cover physiological stress may precipitate hypoadrenalism.
5. Treatment is the same as the acute phase of treatment of hypoadrenal crisis except fluid replacement will not need to be as vigorous.

Waterhouse–Friedrichsen syndrome
1. Haemorrhagic infarction of the adrenal glands may occur as a complication of severe, overwhelming infection.
2. It is associated with severe shock and DIC.
3. Although clinical features similar to those of hypoadrenalism are found there is little evidence of steroid deficiency.
4. Treatment is as for hypoadrenal crisis plus treatment of shock, sepsis and DIC.

Bibliography
Himathongkam T, Newmark SR, Greenfield M, *et al.* Acute adrenal insufficiency. *JAMA* 1974; **230**:1317
Vallotton MB. Endocrine emergencies. Disorders of the adrenal cortex. *Baillieres Clin Endocrinol Metab* 1992; **6**:41

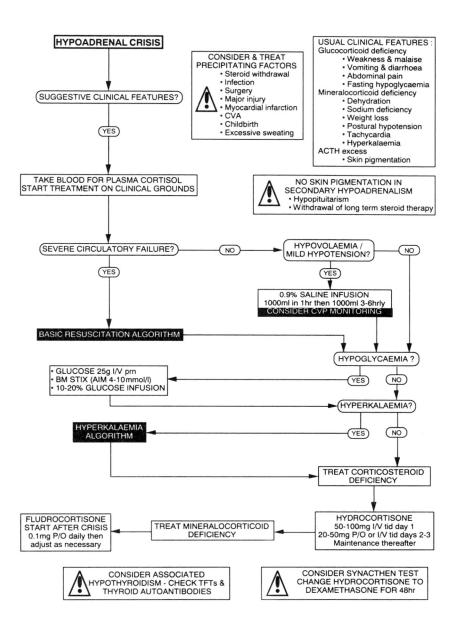

HYPOADRENAL CRISIS

SUGGESTIVE CLINICAL FEATURES?
└ YES

CONSIDER & TREAT
PRECIPITATING FACTORS
- Steroid withdrawal
- Infection
- Surgery
- Major injury
- Myocardial infarction
- CVA
- Childbirth
- Excessive sweating

USUAL CLINICAL FEATURES :
Glucocorticoid deficiency
- Weakness & malaise
- Vomiting & diarrhoea
- Abdominal pain
- Fasting hypoglycaemia
Mineralocorticoid deficiency
- Dehydration
- Sodium deficiency
- Weight loss
- Postural hypotension
- Tachycardia
- Hyperkalaemia
ACTH excess
- Skin pigmentation

TAKE BLOOD FOR PLASMA CORTISOL
START TREATMENT ON CLINICAL GROUNDS

NO SKIN PIGMENTATION IN
SECONDARY HYPOADRENALISM
- Hypopituitarism
- Withdrawal of long term steroid therapy

SEVERE CIRCULATORY FAILURE? ──NO──> HYPOVOLAEMIA /
MILD HYPOTENSION? ──NO──>
└ YES   └ YES

0.9% SALINE INFUSION
1000ml in 1hr then 1000ml 3-6hrly
CONSIDER CVP MONITORING

BASIC RESUSCITATION ALGORITHM

HYPOGLYCAEMIA ?

- GLUCOSE 25g I/V prn
- BM STIX (AIM 4-10 mmol/l)
- 10-20% GLUCOSE INFUSION
<── YES   NO

HYPERKALAEMIA?

HYPERKALAEMIA
ALGORITHM
<── YES   NO

TREAT CORTICOSTEROID
DEFICIENCY

FLUDROCORTISONE
START AFTER CRISIS
0.1mg P/O daily then
adjust as necessary
<── TREAT MINERALOCORTICOID
DEFICIENCY
<── HYDROCORTISONE
50-100mg I/V tid day 1
20-50mg P/O or I/V tid days 2-3
Maintenance thereafter

CONSIDER ASSOCIATED
HYPOTHYROIDISM - CHECK TFTs &
THYROID AUTOANTIBODIES

CONSIDER SYNACTHEN TEST
CHANGE HYDROCORTISONE TO
DEXAMETHASONE FOR 48hr

6.7 Hypopituitary crisis

Clinical features
1. Clinical features are of combined adrenal, thyroid and gonadotrophin hormone deficiencies.
2. Acute hypopituitary crisis is often precipitated by a metabolic stress similar to other endocrine deficiency states.
3. Symptoms have often developed gradually progressing to coma.
4. Mineralocorticoid production is independent of ACTH so is usually normal in pituitary failure; thus potassium levels are not raised.
5. Posterior pituitary involvement may cause diabetes insipidus but polyuria is often masked by steroid deficiency.
6. Conversely, inappropriate ADH secretion may occur with hypothyroidism.

Pituitary function tests
1. Baseline levels of cortisol, thyroxine, ACTH and TSH are low.
2. Baseline measurement of pituitary hormones is all that is required acutely. Dynamic function tests can wait.
3. More sophisticated tests of pituitary function are rarely needed to confirm pituitary crisis.
4. If polyuria occurs diabetes insipidus is likely if plasma osmolality >310 mOsmol/kg and urine osmolality <200 mOsmol/kg.
5. In pituitary apoplexy CT scan will reveal an enlarged sella turcica and parasellar haemorrhage. Lumbar puncture (after excluding raised intracranial pressure) often reveals xanthochromia.

Treatment
1. Replacement of glucocorticoids and correction of hypoglycaemia is urgent.
2. A precipitating cause should be corrected.
3. Replacement of thyroid hormones should not be started before steroid replacement as the increased metabolic rate may worsen the crisis.
4. Diabetes insipidus may require DDAVP replacement. 5% glucose infusions should not be given with DDAVP treatment since the combination may lead to water intoxication, particularly if glucocorticoids are not replaced and plasma osmolality is not monitored.

Bibliography
Edwards CRW, Kitau MJ, Chard T, *et al.* Vasopressin analogue DDAVP in diabetes insipidus. *BMJ* 1973; **3**:375
Gaillard RC. Pituitary gland emergencies. *Baillieres Clin Endocrinol Metab* 1992; **6**:57
Garrod O. Hypopituitary coma. *Hosp Med* 1967; **2**:300
Robinson JL. Sudden blindness in pituitary tumours. *J Neurosurg* 1972; **36**:83

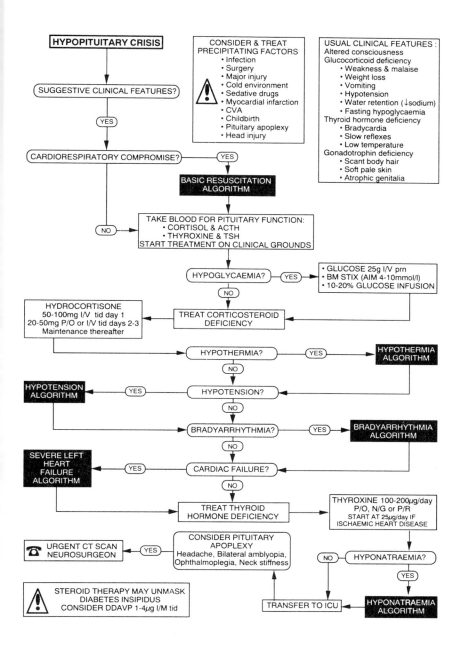

HYPOPITUITARY CRISIS

SUGGESTIVE CLINICAL FEATURES?

YES

CARDIORESPIRATORY COMPROMISE? — YES

NO

CONSIDER & TREAT
PRECIPITATING FACTORS
• Infection
• Surgery
• Major injury
• Cold environment
• Sedative drugs
• Myocardial infarction
• CVA
• Childbirth
• Pituitary apoplexy
• Head injury

USUAL CLINICAL FEATURES :
Altered consciousness
Glucocorticoid deficiency
• Weakness & malaise
• Weight loss
• Vomiting
• Hypotension
• Water retention (↓sodium)
• Fasting hypoglycaemia
Thyroid hormone deficiency
• Bradycardia
• Slow reflexes
• Low temperature
Gonadotrophin deficiency
• Scant body hair
• Soft pale skin
• Atrophic genitalia

BASIC RESUSCITATION
ALGORITHM

TAKE BLOOD FOR PITUITARY FUNCTION:
• CORTISOL & ACTH
• THYROXINE & TSH
START TREATMENT ON CLINICAL GROUNDS

HYPOGLYCAEMIA? — YES

NO

• GLUCOSE 25g I/V prn
• BM STIX (AIM 4-10mmol/l)
• 10-20% GLUCOSE INFUSION

HYDROCORTISONE
50-100mg I/V tid day 1
20-50mg P/O or I/V tid days 2-3
Maintenance thereafter

TREAT CORTICOSTEROID
DEFICIENCY

HYPOTHERMIA? — YES — HYPOTHERMIA
ALGORITHM

NO

HYPOTENSION
ALGORITHM — YES — HYPOTENSION?

NO

BRADYARRHYTHMIA? — YES — BRADYARRHYTHMIA
ALGORITHM

NO

SEVERE LEFT
HEART
FAILURE
ALGORITHM — YES — CARDIAC FAILURE?

NO

TREAT THYROID
HORMONE DEFICIENCY

THYROXINE 100-200µg/day
P/O, N/G or P/R
START AT 25µg/day IF
ISCHAEMIC HEART DISEASE

URGENT CT SCAN
NEUROSURGEON — YES —
CONSIDER PITUITARY
APOPLEXY
Headache, Bilateral amblyopia,
Ophthalmoplegia, Neck stiffness

NO — HYPONATRAEMIA?

YES

STEROID THERAPY MAY UNMASK
DIABETES INSIPIDUS
CONSIDER DDAVP 1-4µg I/M tid

TRANSFER TO ICU

HYPONATRAEMIA
ALGORITHM

7. Gastrointestinal

7.1 Gastrointestinal bleeding

Diagnosis
1. The patient should be adequately resuscitated first.
2. Early endoscopy should be performed for all large bleeds. Therapeutic injection, laser therapy, etc. may prove highly successful.

Stress ulceration
1. The current incidence of significant bleeding (i.e. >2 Units) from stress ulceration is <10% with a direct mortality less than 1–2%, whether the patient is receiving prophylaxis or not.
2. H_2 antagonists (or proton pump inhibitors) ± antacids to keep pH ≥5 are usually effective in stopping bleeding from stress ulceration once it occurs. Surgery is very rarely necessary.

Management
1. CVP ± PA catheter monitoring may be useful, especially in the elderly and those with cardiac dysfunction. Caution should be exercised as clotting abnormalities are often present.
2. Colloid is a better volume expander than blood. Shocked patients should receive a combination, particularly as most stored blood is plasma deplete.
3. Coagulopathies should be actively corrected.
4. Platelet transfusions should be given—despite normal levels—if aspirin has been ingested recently as platelet function may be affected.
5. H_2 antagonists, omeprazole and antacids will not generally stop bleeding from non-stress ulcers though they do facilitate ulcer healing.
6. Unless varices are present, a N/G tube should be inserted to give medication and assess the rate of bleeding.

Surgery
1. Surgeons should remain well-informed throughout.
2. Mortality is significantly higher in massive or recurrent bleeding. Early surgery should be considered in these cases.
3. Early surgery should be considered in the elderly.

Lower G-I bleeding
1. Endoscopy, isotope scanning and angiography may delineate the site of the lesion. Angiography will only reveal a lesion if there is active bleeding of at least 0.5 ml/min.
2. Early surgery is the preferred treatment for massive lower G-I bleeding.

Bibliography
Boley SJ, Brandt LJ, Frank MS. Severe lower intestinal bleeding: Diagnosis and treatment. *Clin Gastroenterol* 1981; **10**: 65
Chung SC, Leung JW, Steele RJ, Lia K. Endoscopic injection of adrenaline for actively bleeding ulcers. *BMJ* 1988; **296**: 1631
Lacroix J, Infante-Rivard C, Jenicek M, Gauthier M. Prophylaxis of upper gastrointestinal bleeding in intensive care units. A meta-analysis. *Crit Care Med* 1989; **17**: 862
Laurence BH, Cotton PB. Bleeding gastroduodenal ulcers: Non-operative management. *World J Surg* 1987; **11**: 295

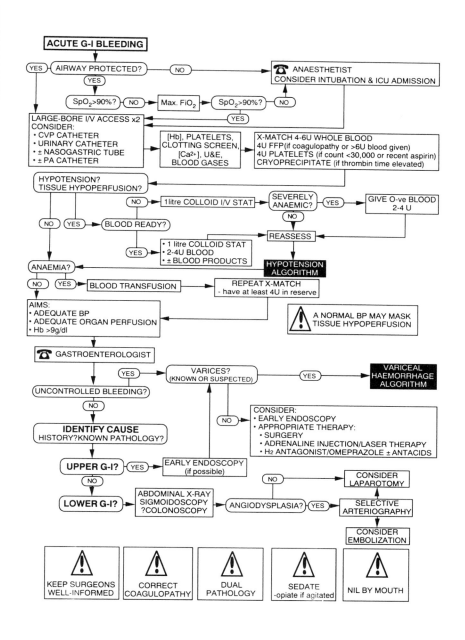

ACUTE G-I BLEEDING

Laurence BH. Acute gastrointestinal bleeding. In: Oh TE (Ed.) Intensive care manual. 3rd edition. Butterworths, Sydney, 1990, p219

Leicester RJ. Gastrointestinal haemorrhage. *Medicine International* 1990; **77**: 3188

Wilcox CM, Spenney JG. Stress ulcer prophylaxis in medical patients: who, what and how much? *Am J Gastroenterol* 1988; **83**: 1199

7.2 Acute variceal haemorrhage

General
1. Acute variceal bleeding occurs in a third of cirrhotic patients.
2. Rebleeding occurs in 75% of those who survive the first bleed.
3. >30% of cases of upper G-I bleeding in cirrhotics have a non-variceal origin. Dual pathology should also be considered.

Sclerotherapy
1. Sclerotherapy is the current treatment of choice; it arrests bleeding in over 80% of cases and reduces early rebleeding.
2. Early therapeutic endoscopy and sclerotherapy should be performed by an experienced operator. If such facilities are not readily available then insertion of a Sengstaken-type tube for balloon tamponade should be considered for significant bleeds.

Sengstaken-type tubes (Sengstaken–Blakemore, Minnesota...)
1. A Sengstaken-type tube should be inserted for large variceal bleeds.
2. The oesophageal balloon should not be inflated initially. Compression of the gastric balloon on the cardia (and fundus) should control bleeding satisfactorily in most cases. Adequate traction of the tube should be maintained (approx. 1 kg weight). If oesophageal balloon inflation is necessary (after confirmation of correct positioning of tube), deflate at hrly intervals to avoid pressure necrosis.
3. Continuous aspiration of the oesophageal lumen of tube reduces the risk of aspiration.

Other therapies
1. Vasopressin acts by reducing portal blood flow and causing splanchnic vasoconstriction. It will only control bleeding temporarily in 60% of cases. Simultaneous administration of GTN (by patch or I/V infusion) may reduce side-effects.
2. Somatostatin is a selective splanchnic vasoconstrictor and reduces portal blood flow and collateral blood flow in portal hypertension. It is well tolerated and initial control of bleeding is reasonable.
3. Octreotide is also being investigated; preliminary data suggest an efficacy comparable to balloon tamponade.
4. Staplegun transection or transjugular portal shunt or open porto-caval shunt should be considered when repeated sclerotherapy proves unsuccessful.
5. β-blockade has been used as secondary prophylaxis.

Bibliography
Burroughs AK, Hamilton G, Phillips A, *et al*. A comparison of sclerotherapy with staple transection for the emergency control of bleeding from esophageal varices. *N Engl J Med* 1989; **321**: 857
Burroughs AK, McCormack PA, Hughes MD, *et al*. Randomised double-blind placebo controlled trial of somatostatin for variceal bleeding. *Gastroenterology* 1990; **99**: 1388
Gimson AE, Westaby D, Hegarty J, *et al*. A randomized trial of vasopressin and vasopressin plus nitroglycerine in the control of acute variceal haemorrhage. *Hepatology* 1986; **6**: 410
Hayes PC, Davis JM, Lewis JA, Bouchier IAD. Meta-analysis of value of propranolol in prevention of variceal haemorrhage. *Lancet* 1990; **ii**: 153
McKee R. A study of octreotide in oesophageal varices. *Digestion* 1990; **45** (Suppl): 60

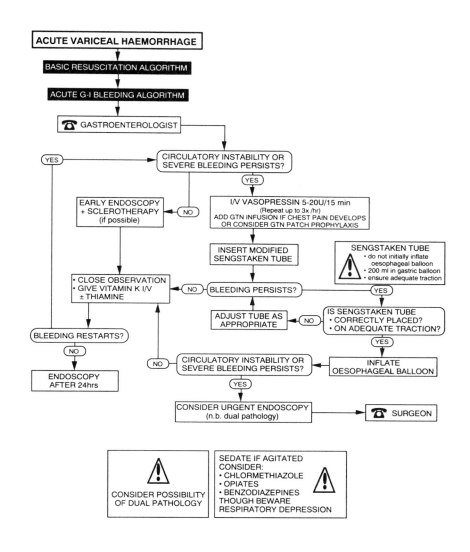

ACUTE VARICEAL HAEMORRHAGE

BASIC RESUSCITATION ALGORITHM

ACUTE G-I BLEEDING ALGORITHM

☎ GASTROENTEROLOGIST

CIRCULATORY INSTABILITY OR
SEVERE BLEEDING PERSISTS?

YES

YES

I/V VASOPRESSIN 5-20U/15 min
(Repeat up to 3x /hr)
ADD GTN INFUSION IF CHEST PAIN DEVELOPS
OR CONSIDER GTN PATCH PROPHYLAXIS

NO

EARLY ENDOSCOPY
+ SCLEROTHERAPY
(if possible)

INSERT MODIFIED
SENGSTAKEN TUBE

SENGSTAKEN TUBE
⚠ • do not initially inflate
   oesophageal balloon
 • 200 ml in gastric balloon
 • ensure adequate traction

• CLOSE OBSERVATION
• GIVE VITAMIN K I/V
  ± THIAMINE

NO BLEEDING PERSISTS? YES

ADJUST TUBE AS
APPROPRIATE

NO

IS SENGSTAKEN TUBE
• CORRECTLY PLACED?
• ON ADEQUATE TRACTION?

BLEEDING RESTARTS?

NO

YES

ENDOSCOPY
AFTER 24hrs

NO CIRCULATORY INSTABILITY OR
SEVERE BLEEDING PERSISTS?

INFLATE
OESOPHAGEAL BALLOON

YES

CONSIDER URGENT ENDOSCOPY
(n.b. dual pathology)

☎ SURGEON

⚠

CONSIDER POSSIBILITY
OF DUAL PATHOLOGY

SEDATE IF AGITATED
CONSIDER:
• CHLORMETHIAZOLE
• OPIATES
• BENZODIAZEPINES
THOUGH BEWARE
RESPIRATORY DEPRESSION ⚠

Poynard T, Cales P, Pasta L, *et al.* Beta-adrenergic antagonist drugs in the prevention of gastrointestinal bleeding in patients with cirrhosis and esophageal varices: an analysis of data and prognostic factors in 589 patients from four randomized clinical trials. *N Engl J Med* 1991; **324**: 1532

Westaby D, Hayes PC, Gimson AES, Polson RJ, Williams R. Controlled clinical trial of injection sclerotherapy for active variceal bleeding. *Hepatology* 1989; **9**: 274

Vlavianos P, Gimson AES, Westaby D, Williams R. Balloon tamponade in variceal bleeding: use and misuse. *BMJ* 1989; **298**: 1158

7.3 Acute abdominal pain

Causes

1. There are many causes of abdominal pain including mucosal irritation (e.g. gastritis), smooth muscle spasm (e.g. renal and biliary colic, enterocolitis), capsular stretching (e.g. enlarged liver, spleen), peritoneal inflammation and referred 'medical' causes (e.g. MI, diabetes).
2. A careful history and examination should be performed assessing the character, duration and frequency of pain, location and distribution, and aggravating/relieving factors (e.g. meals, posture).
3. Surgical causes of acute abdominal pain should be excluded before diagnosing a 'medical' cause e.g. diabetes.
4. Acute pancreatitis may occur in the absence of a raised amylase.
5. Ischaemic colitis often presents with abdominal pain and bloody diarrhoea. A very tender abdomen, increasing metabolic acidosis (despite adequate resuscitation) and the presence of dilated, widely separated bowel loops with 'thumb printing' suggestive of mucosal oedema on abdominal X-ray are also suggestive of ischaemic or infarcted bowel. Laparotomy ± prior angiography is indicated. However, ischaemic colitis may also present without abdominal tenderness; diagnosis is difficult and a high index of suspicion should be harboured.
6. Pregnancy must be excluded in any woman of child-bearing age presenting with lower abdominal pain.

Laparotomy

1. Surgery is usually indicated when there is:
   - rupture/perforation of an organ
   - generalized peritonitis
   - localized peritonitis (depending on cause)
   - mechanical bowel obstruction
2. Laparotomy may sometimes be avoided by laparoscopic or radiological procedures (e.g. drainage of abscesses).
3. The patient should be adequately resuscitated first.

Fictitious pain

1. Suspect if history of multiple operations in numerous hospitals.
2. Suspect if inconsistent history or examination findings.
3. Suspect if severity of symptoms out of proportion to other signs e.g. heart rate, blood pressure. Such patients may often hyperventilate and sweat profusely.
4. Look closely for injection sites suggesting history of intravenous drug taking.

Bibliography

Hawthorn IE. Abdominal pain as a cause of acute admission to hospital. *J R Coll Surg Edinb* 1992; **37**: 389

Lerch MM, Riehl J, Buechsel R, *et al.* Bedside ultrasound in decision making for emergency surgery: its role in medical intensive care patients. *Am J Emerg Med* 1992; **10**: 35

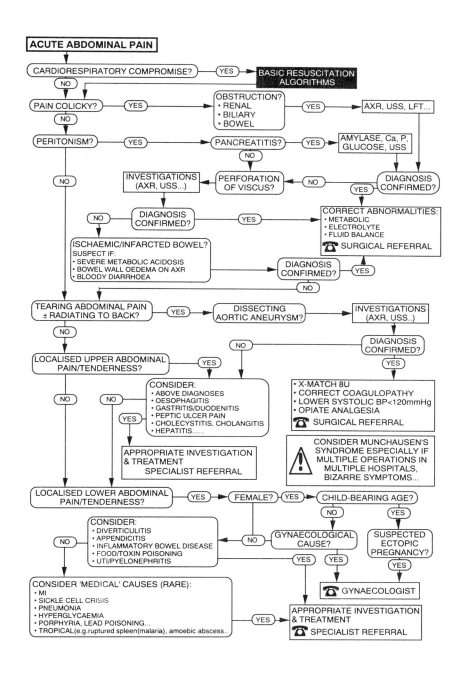

ACUTE ABDOMINAL PAIN

CARDIORESPIRATORY COMPROMISE? — YES → **BASIC RESUSCITATION ALGORITHMS**

NO

PAIN COLICKY? — YES → OBSTRUCTION?
- RENAL
- BILIARY
- BOWEL
— YES → AXR, USS, LFT...

NO

PERITONISM? — YES → PANCREATITIS? — YES → AMYLASE, Ca, P, GLUCOSE, USS

NO

NO

INVESTIGATIONS (AXR, USS...) ← PERFORATION OF VISCUS? ← NO ← DIAGNOSIS CONFIRMED?

YES

NO → DIAGNOSIS CONFIRMED? — YES → CORRECT ABNORMALITIES:
- METABOLIC
- ELECTROLYTE
- FLUID BALANCE
☎ SURGICAL REFERRAL

ISCHAEMIC/INFARCTED BOWEL?
SUSPECT IF:
- SEVERE METABOLIC ACIDOSIS
- BOWEL WALL OEDEMA ON AXR
- BLOODY DIARRHOEA
→ DIAGNOSIS CONFIRMED? — YES

NO

TEARING ABDOMINAL PAIN ± RADIATING TO BACK? — YES → DISSECTING AORTIC ANEURYSM? → INVESTIGATIONS (AXR, USS..)

NO

NO → DIAGNOSIS CONFIRMED?

LOCALISED UPPER ABDOMINAL PAIN/TENDERNESS? — YES

YES

NO   NO → CONSIDER:
- ABOVE DIAGNOSES
- OESOPHAGITIS
- GASTRITIS/DUODENITIS
- PEPTIC ULCER PAIN
- CHOLECYSTITIS, CHOLANGITIS
- HEPATITIS......

YES

- X-MATCH 8U
- CORRECT COAGULOPATHY
- LOWER SYSTOLIC BP<120mmHg
- OPIATE ANALGESIA
☎ SURGICAL REFERRAL

APPROPRIATE INVESTIGATION & TREATMENT
SPECIALIST REFERRAL

⚠ CONSIDER MUNCHAUSEN'S SYNDROME ESPECIALLY IF MULTIPLE OPERATIONS IN MULTIPLE HOSPITALS, BIZARRE SYMPTOMS...

LOCALISED LOWER ABDOMINAL PAIN/TENDERNESS? — YES → FEMALE? — YES → CHILD-BEARING AGE?

NO   YES

CONSIDER:
- DIVERTICULITIS
- APPENDICITIS
- INFLAMMATORY BOWEL DISEASE
- FOOD/TOXIN POISONING
- UTI/PYELONEPHRITIS
← NO ← GYNAECOLOGICAL CAUSE?

SUSPECTED ECTOPIC PREGNANCY?

NO

YES   YES

YES

CONSIDER 'MEDICAL' CAUSES (RARE):
- MI
- SICKLE CELL CRISIS
- PNEUMONIA
- HYPERGLYCAEMIA
- PORPHYRIA, LEAD POISONING...
- TROPICAL(e.g.ruptured spleen(malaria), amoebic abscess..
— YES → APPROPRIATE INVESTIGATION & TREATMENT
☎ SPECIALIST REFERRAL

☎ GYNAECOLOGIST

7.4 Severe vomiting

General
1. Vomiting is a symptom of many disease processes ranging from pain to gastrointenstinal irritation and obstruction. Aim to identify and treat the cause promptly.

Management
1. Ensure adequate hydration and electrolyte replacement. Acid loss may result in hypochloraemia, hyponatraemia, hypokalaemia, and metabolic alkalosis.
2. Give drugs parenterally or per rectum to ensure absorption.
3. If vomiting is prolonged, consider enteral nutrition via a naso-jejunal tube or jejunostomy if distal obstruction is ruled out. Alternatively, parenteral nutrition should be considered in the presence of pancreatitis or bowel pathology.
4. Stop drugs known to have irritant effects on the gastrointestinal tract e.g. NSAIDs.
5. Continuous nasogastric drainage should be used if bowel obstruction or paralytic ileus is present as gastric distension is a powerful stimulus for vomiting and the risk of aspiration pneumonia is lessened.

Anti-emetics
1. The oral route should be initially avoided until symptoms have been brought under control.
2. Metoclopramide aids gastric emptying in addition to its centrally-acting effects.
3. Both metoclopramide and prochlorperazine may induce extra-pyramidal side-effects e.g. oculogyric crises.
4. Antihistamines and phenothiazines may cause excessive sedation.

Cause	First-line agent
Central	hyoscine
e.g. Ménière's disease,	antihistamines e.g. promethazine
motion sickness, labyrinthitis	prochlorperazine
and positional vertigo	
Paralytic ileus	metoclopramide
Delayed gastric emptying	
Acute abdomen	
Metabolic	cyclizine
	metoclopramide
Drug-induced	prochlorperazine
e.g. cytotoxics	ondansetron
	domperidone

Bibliography
Gralla RJ. Current issues in the management of nausea and vomiting. *Ann Oncol* 1993; **4** (Suppl.3) S3
Rowbotham DJ. Current management of postoperative nausea and vomiting. *Br J Anaesth* 1992; **69** (Suppl.1) 46S

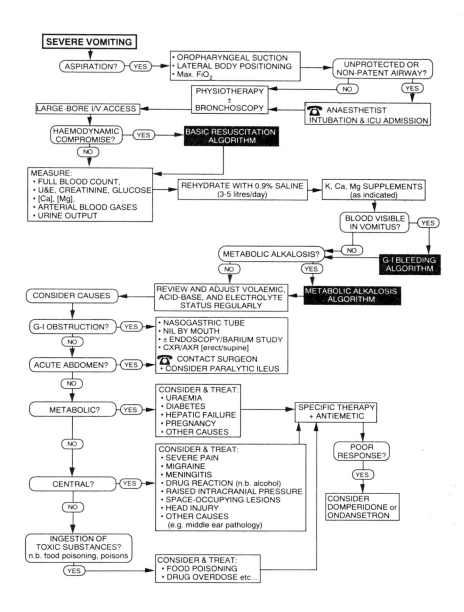

SEVERE VOMITING

ASPIRATION? — YES → • OROPHARYNGEAL SUCTION / • LATERAL BODY POSITIONING / • Max. FiO$_2$ → UNPROTECTED OR NON-PATENT AIRWAY?

UNPROTECTED OR NON-PATENT AIRWAY? — NO → PHYSIOTHERAPY ± BRONCHOSCOPY

UNPROTECTED OR NON-PATENT AIRWAY? — YES → ☎ ANAESTHETIST INTUBATION & ICU ADMISSION

LARGE-BORE I/V ACCESS

HAEMODYNAMIC COMPROMISE? — YES → **BASIC RESUSCITATION ALGORITHM**

HAEMODYNAMIC COMPROMISE? — NO →

MEASURE:
• FULL BLOOD COUNT,
• U&E, CREATININE, GLUCOSE
• [Ca], [Mg],
• ARTERIAL BLOOD GASES
• URINE OUTPUT

→ REHYDRATE WITH 0.9% SALINE (3-5 litres/day) → K, Ca, Mg SUPPLEMENTS (as indicated)

BLOOD VISIBLE IN VOMITUS? — YES → **G-I BLEEDING ALGORITHM**

BLOOD VISIBLE IN VOMITUS? — NO →

METABOLIC ALKALOSIS? — NO →
METABOLIC ALKALOSIS? — YES → **METABOLIC ALKALOSIS ALGORITHM**

REVIEW AND ADJUST VOLAEMIC, ACID-BASE, AND ELECTROLYTE STATUS REGULARLY

CONSIDER CAUSES

G-I OBSTRUCTION? — YES → • NASOGASTRIC TUBE / • NIL BY MOUTH / • ± ENDOSCOPY/BARIUM STUDY / • CXR/AXR [erect/supine] / ☎ CONTACT SURGEON / • CONSIDER PARALYTIC ILEUS

G-I OBSTRUCTION? — NO →

ACUTE ABDOMEN? — YES →

ACUTE ABDOMEN? — NO →

METABOLIC? — YES → CONSIDER & TREAT:
• URAEMIA
• DIABETES
• HEPATIC FAILURE
• PREGNANCY
• OTHER CAUSES
→ SPECIFIC THERAPY + ANTIEMETIC

METABOLIC? — NO →

CENTRAL? — YES → CONSIDER & TREAT:
• SEVERE PAIN
• MIGRAINE
• MENINGITIS
• DRUG REACTION (n.b. alcohol)
• RAISED INTRACRANIAL PRESSURE
• SPACE-OCCUPYING LESIONS
• HEAD INJURY
• OTHER CAUSES
  (e.g. middle ear pathology)

CENTRAL? — NO →

SPECIFIC THERAPY + ANTIEMETIC → POOR RESPONSE? — YES → CONSIDER DOMPERIDONE or ONDANSETRON

INGESTION OF TOXIC SUBSTANCES? n.b. food poisoning, poisons — YES → CONSIDER & TREAT:
• FOOD POISONING
• DRUG OVERDOSE etc...

7.5 Severe diarrhoea

General

1. Take a careful history including duration, contacts, foreign travel, presence of blood, drug/toxin ingestion, associated symptoms.
2. Ensure adequate hydration and electrolyte replacement (including potassium and magnesium).
3. Ischaemic colitis often presents with abdominal pain and bloody diarrhoea though the blood may not be obvious macroscopically. A very tender abdomen, increasing metabolic acidosis (despite adequate resuscitation) and the presence of dilated, widely separated bowel loops with 'thumb printing' suggestive of mucosal oedema on abdominal X-ray are also suggestive of ischaemic or infarcted bowel. Laparotomy ± prior angiography is indicated. However, ischaemic colitis may also present without abdominal tenderness; diagnosis is difficult and a high index of suspicion should be harboured.
4. Enteral nutrition is rarely the sole cause of diarrhoea—concurrent use of antibiotics are more often responsible.

Infective diarrhoea

1. Antibiotics for infective diarrhoea should be avoided unless indicated for specific conditions e.g. metronidazole for amoebic dysentry, chloramphenicol or ampicillin for typhoid, tetracycline for cholera . . .
2. Consider *Clostridium difficile* infection if diarrhoea acquired in hospital or closed communities.
3. Cholestyramine may reduce diarrhoea in *C.difficile* infection by binding the toxin.
4. Avoid anti-diarrhoeal agents in infective diarrhoea.

Gastrointestinal malabsorption

1. Diarrhoea may be a symptom of gastrointestinal malabsorption in association with steatorrhoea, weight loss, oedema and anaemia.
2. *Causes include:*
   • coeliac disease (gluten-enteropathy)
   • chronic pancreatitis
   • tropical sprue
   • post-surgical intestinal hurry (e.g. post-vagotomy)
   • infections (e.g. giardiasis, strongyloidiasis)
   • causes of obstructive jaundice
   • bacterial overgrowth

Inflammatory bowel disease

1. Ulcerative colitis usually presents as bloody diarrhoea while Crohn's disease more commonly presents with non-bloody diarrhoea, fever and abdominal pain. In ulcerative colitis blood and mucus passed per rectum with an otherwise formed stool suggests rectal involvement only while diarrhoea suggests more extensive disease.
2. Diagnostic investigations for ulcerative colitis and Crohn's disease are generally similar, involving sigmoidoscopy and biopsy, and radiological studies.
3. For severe disease specialist advice should be sought urgently. Treatment usually consists of systemic and topical corticosteroids, 5-amino salicylic acid, rehydration, transfusion (if necessary), adequate nutrition (low residue enteral or parenteral), including iron, folate, and vitamin replacement.

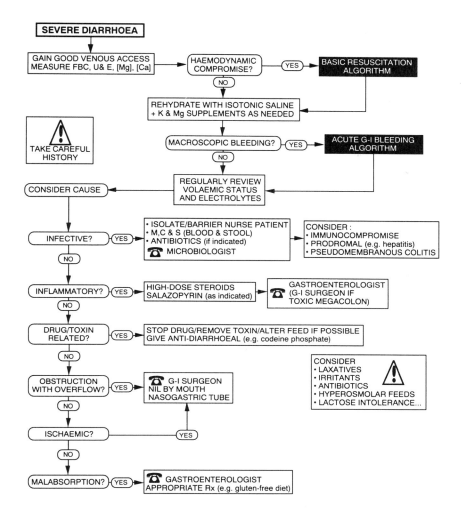

4. Surgery is indicated in ulcerative colitis for toxic megacolon, bowel perforation, and deterioration despite optimal medical treatment. In Crohn's disease surgery should be considered when there is obstruction, abscess or fistula formation.
5. Anti-diarrhoeal drugs should generally be avoided.

Bibliography
Chak A, Banwell JG. Traveler's diarrhea. Gastroenterol *Clin North Am* 1993; **22**: 549
Nathwani D, Wood MJ. The management of travellers' diarrhoea. *J Antimicrob Chemother* 1993; **31**: 623
Park SI, Giannella RA. Approach to the adult patient with acute diarrhea. *Gastroenterol Clin North Am* 1993; **22**: 483
Wolf DC, Giannella RA. Antibiotic therapy for bacterial enterocolitis: a comprehensive review. *Am J Gastroenterol* 1993; **88**: 1667

7.6/7.7 Hepatic failure

General
1. Viral hepatitis and paracetamol are the commonest causes of acute liver failure.
2. N-acetylcysteine appears effective up to 36 hr after paracetamol ingestion.
3. N-acetylcysteine improves oxygen delivery and consumption in patients with both paracetamol-induced fulminant hepatic failure and in FHF from other causes.

Encephalopathy and cerebral oedema
1. Early administration of lactulose may be beneficial in early encephalopathy.
2. Mortality is much higher for Grades III–IV encephalopathy.
3. Cerebral oedema is much commoner for Grades III–IV (75% with Grade IV). ICP monitoring in a specialist centre is indicated.
4. Avoid hypotension, hypoxaemia, and hypercapnia.
5. Steroids are ineffective.

Renal failure
1. Occurs in 30–75% of Grade IV encephalopathy and is commoner with paracetamol.
2. Consider hypovolaemia, hypotension and nephrotoxic drugs.
3. High dose frusemide should not be given and care should be taken with high dose mannitol.
4. With renal replacement (especially dialysis) care is needed to avoid hypovolaemia or too rapid removal of solute because of the risk of cerebral oedema.

Metabolic
1. Hypoglycaemia is very common. Monitor hourly. Give 20–50% glucose if necessary.
2. Both metabolic alkalosis and acidosis can occur. Correct hypokalaemia.

Cardiorespiratory
1. Arrhythmias are common. Obvious causes should be corrected e.g. hypokalaemia.
2. Hypoxaemia is common and may be caused by ventilation–perfusion mismatch due to shunting, infection, aspiration, etc.

Sepsis
1. The patient in fulminant hepatic failure is immunocompromised.
2. Regular cultures are essential.
3. Antibiotics and antifungals should be considered in recovering patients in whom improvement in prothrombin time ceases.

Transplantation
1. Early discussion should take place with a specialist centre.
2. Important factors for consideration: age, aetiology, interval between jaundice and encephalopathy, bilirubin (>300 µmol/l) and prothrombin time (>50 sec).

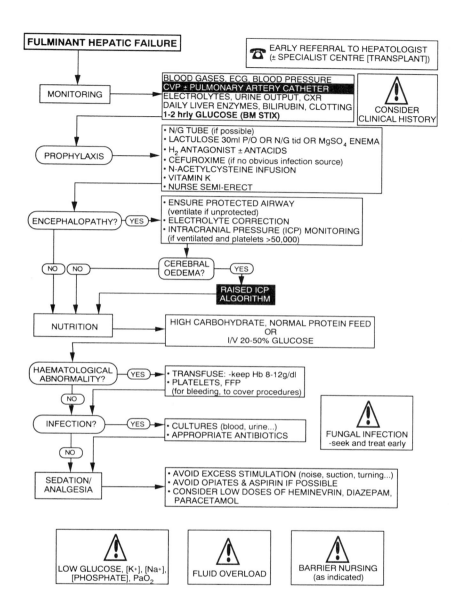

FULMINANT HEPATIC FAILURE

☎ EARLY REFERRAL TO HEPATOLOGIST
(± SPECIALIST CENTRE [TRANSPLANT])

MONITORING →

BLOOD GASES, ECG, BLOOD PRESSURE
CVP ± PULMONARY ARTERY CATHETER
ELECTROLYTES, URINE OUTPUT, CXR
DAILY LIVER ENZYMES, BILIRUBIN, CLOTTING
1-2 hrly GLUCOSE (BM STIX)

⚠ CONSIDER CLINICAL HISTORY

PROPHYLAXIS →
• N/G TUBE (if possible)
• LACTULOSE 30ml P/O OR N/G tid OR MgSO₄ ENEMA
• H₂ ANTAGONIST ± ANTACIDS
• CEFUROXIME (if no obvious infection source)
• N-ACETYLCYSTEINE INFUSION
• VITAMIN K
• NURSE SEMI-ERECT

ENCEPHALOPATHY? —YES→
• ENSURE PROTECTED AIRWAY
(ventilate if unprotected)
• ELECTROLYTE CORRECTION
• INTRACRANIAL PRESSURE (ICP) MONITORING
(if ventilated and platelets >50,000)

NO NO → CEREBRAL OEDEMA? —YES→

RAISED ICP ALGORITHM

NUTRITION →
HIGH CARBOHYDRATE, NORMAL PROTEIN FEED
OR
I/V 20-50% GLUCOSE

HAEMATOLOGICAL ABNORMALITY? —YES→
• TRANSFUSE: -keep Hb 8-12g/dl
• PLATELETS, FFP
(for bleeding, to cover procedures)

NO

INFECTION? —YES→
• CULTURES (blood, urine...)
• APPROPRIATE ANTIBIOTICS

⚠ FUNGAL INFECTION
-seek and treat early

NO

SEDATION/ ANALGESIA →
• AVOID EXCESS STIMULATION (noise, suction, turning...)
• AVOID OPIATES & ASPIRIN IF POSSIBLE
• CONSIDER LOW DOSES OF HEMINEVRIN, DIAZEPAM, PARACETAMOL

⚠ LOW GLUCOSE, [K+], [Na+], [PHOSPHATE], PaO₂

⚠ FLUID OVERLOAD

⚠ BARRIER NURSING (as indicated)

Acute on chronic liver failure

1. Ascites is far commoner. Infected ascites should be ruled out as a cause of decompensation.
2. Other causes of G-I bleeding other than varices e.g. peptic ulcer should be considered.
3. Neomycin may be useful for a few days only to reduce breakdown of gastrointestinal blood.

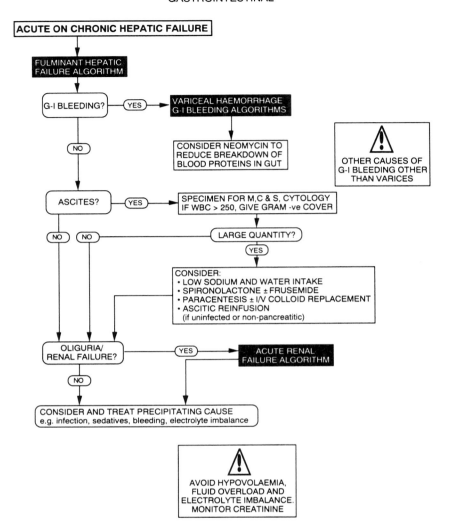

ACUTE ON CHRONIC HEPATIC FAILURE

FULMINANT HEPATIC
FAILURE ALGORITHM

G-I BLEEDING? — YES → VARICEAL HAEMORRHAGE
G-I BLEEDING ALGORITHMS

NO

CONSIDER NEOMYCIN TO
REDUCE BREAKDOWN OF
BLOOD PROTEINS IN GUT

⚠ OTHER CAUSES OF
G-I BLEEDING OTHER
THAN VARICES

ASCITES? — YES → SPECIMEN FOR M,C & S, CYTOLOGY
IF WBC > 250, GIVE GRAM -ve COVER

NO   NO — LARGE QUANTITY?
YES

CONSIDER:
• LOW SODIUM AND WATER INTAKE
• SPIRONOLACTONE ± FRUSEMIDE
• PARACENTESIS ± I/V COLLOID REPLACEMENT
• ASCITIC REINFUSION
  (if uninfected or non-pancreatitic)

OLIGURIA/
RENAL FAILURE? — YES → ACUTE RENAL
FAILURE ALGORITHM

NO

CONSIDER AND TREAT PRECIPITATING CAUSE
e.g. infection, sedatives, bleeding, electrolyte imbalance

⚠ AVOID HYPOVOLAEMIA,
FLUID OVERLOAD AND
ELECTROLYTE IMBALANCE.
MONITOR CREATININE

Bibliography

Harrison PM, Keays R, Bray GP, Alexander GJM, Williams R. Improved outcome of paracetamol-induced fulminant hepatic failure by late administration of acetylcysteine. *Lancet* 1990; **i**:1572

Harrison PM, Wendon JA, Gimson AES, Alexander GJM, Williams R. Improvement by acetylcysteine of hemodynamics and oxygen transport in fulminant hepatic failure. *N Engl J Med* 1991; **324**:1852

Mutimer D, Neuberger J. Acute liver failure: improving outcome despite a paucity of treatment options. *Quart J Med* 1993; **86**:409

Stoller JK. As the liver goes, so goes the lung. *Chest* 1990; **97**:1028

Williams R. Acute liver failure: an overview. In: Vincent JL (Ed.) Update in intensive care & emergency medicine No.8. Springer-Verlag, Berlin, 1989, p376

Notes

8. Neurological

8.1 The unconscious patient

Clinical features

1. Coma is a state of unconsciousness from which the patient cannot be aroused. It should be distinguished from the 'locked in' syndrome and psychogenic unresponsiveness.
2. Patients with the 'locked in' syndrome are aware but cannot respond to stimuli except perhaps by vertical eye movements and blinking.
3. Psychogenic unresponsiveness can be distinguished by the following features:
   • voluntary eye closure
   • resistance to eye opening
   • corneal reflexes present
   • nystagmus in response to cold caloric stimulus
   • normally responsive EEG
4. Loss of consciousness due to metabolic encephalopathy is often preceded by confusion and a progressive deterioration in consciousness and is associated with tremor and/or asterixis and myoclonus.
5. Coma may be caused by conditions associated with severe hypoxaemia but hypoxaemia may be due to ventilatory failure caused by coma.
6. Circulatory failure may cause coma but vasomotor paresis associated with coma may cause severe hypotension requiring fluid and possibly vasopressor therapy.

Monitoring coma

1. Prognosis can be judged from the patient's posture, pupillary and oculovestibular reflexes.
2. Poor prognosis is associated with:
   • decerebrate posturing and rigidity for >24 hr in non-trauma patients
   • decerebrate posturing and rigidity for >2 weeks in trauma patients
   • absent oculovestibular reflexes for >24 hr
   • absent pupillary reflexes for >24 hr in post-anoxic brain injury patients
   • absent pupillary reflexes for >3 days for other patients
3. Hypoxaemia, shock, adrenergic hyperactivity, drug effects and lesions of the 2nd and 3rd cranial nerves must be excluded before interpreting ocular and pupillary reflexes.
4. The Glasgow Coma Scale is a common technique for monitoring the progress of coma producing a score from 15 (normal) to 3 (deep coma):

Eyes open	Score	Best motor response	Score	Best verbal response	Score
Spontaneously	4	Obeys command	6	Orientated	5
To command	3	Localizes pain	5	Disorientated	4
To pain	2	Flexion withdrawal to pain	4	Inappropriate words	3
No response	1	Abnormal flexion to pain	3	Incomprehensible sounds	2
		Extension to pain	2	No response	1
		No response	1		

5. Prognosis deteriorates with duration of coma; patients with post-anoxic coma for 3 days rarely survive without severe disability.

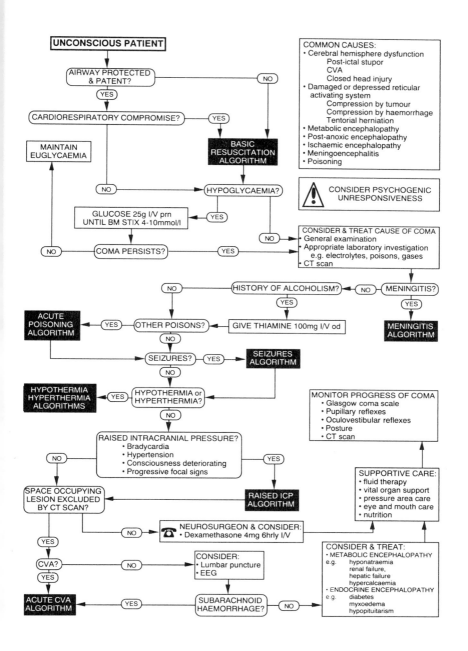

UNCONSCIOUS PATIENT

AIRWAY PROTECTED & PATENT? → NO

YES

CARDIORESPIRATORY COMPROMISE? → YES

MAINTAIN EUGLYCAEMIA

BASIC RESUSCITATION ALGORITHM

COMMON CAUSES:
- Cerebral hemisphere dysfunction
  - Post-ictal stupor
  - CVA
  - Closed head injury
- Damaged or depressed reticular activating system
  - Compression by tumour
  - Compression by haemorrhage
  - Tentorial herniation
- Metabolic encephalopathy
- Post-anoxic encephalopathy
- Ischaemic encephalopathy
- Meningoencephalitis
- Poisoning

CONSIDER PSYCHOGENIC UNRESPONSIVENESS

NO → HYPOGLYCAEMIA?

GLUCOSE 25g I/V prn UNTIL BM STIX 4-10mmol/l → YES

NO → COMA PERSISTS? → YES

NO

CONSIDER & TREAT CAUSE OF COMA
- General examination
- Appropriate laboratory investigation e.g. electrolytes, poisons, gases
- CT scan

NO → HISTORY OF ALCOHOLISM? → NO → MENINGITIS?

YES

YES

ACUTE POISONING ALGORITHM ← YES ← OTHER POISONS? ← GIVE THIAMINE 100mg I/V od

MENINGITIS ALGORITHM

NO

SEIZURES? → YES → SEIZURES ALGORITHM

NO

HYPOTHERMIA HYPERTHERMIA ALGORITHMS ← YES ← HYPOTHERMIA or HYPERTHERMIA?

NO

MONITOR PROGRESS OF COMA
- Glasgow coma scale
- Pupillary reflexes
- Oculovestibular reflexes
- Posture
- CT scan

RAISED INTRACRANIAL PRESSURE?
- Bradycardia
- Hypertension
- Consciousness deteriorating
- Progressive focal signs

NO

YES

RAISED ICP ALGORITHM

SUPPORTIVE CARE:
- fluid therapy
- vital organ support
- pressure area care
- eye and mouth care
- nutrition

SPACE OCCUPYING LESION EXCLUDED BY CT SCAN?

NO → ☎ NEUROSURGEON & CONSIDER:
- Dexamethasone 4mg 6hrly I/V

YES

CVA? → NO

CONSIDER:
- Lumbar puncture
- EEG

YES

CONSIDER & TREAT:
- METABOLIC ENCEPHALOPATHY
  e.g. hyponatraemia
       renal failure
       hepatic failure
       hypercalcaemia
- ENDOCRINE ENCEPHALOPATHY
  e.g. diabetes
       myxoedema
       hypopituitarism

ACUTE CVA ALGORITHM ← YES ← SUBARACHNOID HAEMORRHAGE? → NO

Bibliography

Bates D, Caronna TJ, Cratlidge NEF, *et al.* Prospective study of non-traumatic coma: methods and results in 310 patients. *Ann Neurol* 1977; **2**:211

Brennan RW. Resuscitation from metabolic coma and encephalitis. *Crit Care Med* 1978; **6**:277

Cold GE, Jensen FT, Malmros R. The cerebrovascular CO_2 reactivity during the acute phase of brain injury. *Acta Anesthesiol Scand* 1977; **21**:222

Cold GE, Jensen FT , Malmros R. The effects of $PaCO_2$ reduction on regional cerebral blood flow in the acute phase of brain injury. *Acta Anesthesiol Scand* 1977; **21**:359

Dearden NM, Gibson JS, McDowall DG, *et al.* Effect of high-dose dexamethasone on outcome from severe head injury. *J Neurosurg* 1986; **64**:81

Hanley DF. Coma, intracranial pressure, intensive care, head injury and neoplasia. *Curr Opin Neurol Neurosurg* 1992; **5**:795

Obrist WD, Langfitt TW, Jaggi JL, *et al.* Cerebral blood flow and metabolism in comatose patients with acute head injury: relationship with intracranial hypertension. *J Neurosurg* 1984; **61**:241

Samuels MA. A practical approach to coma diagnosis in the unresponsive patient. *Cleve Clin J Med* 1992; **59**:257

Teasdale G, Jennett B. Assessment of coma and impaired consciousness. A practical scale. *Lancet* 1974; **ii**:81

Notes

8.2 Acute weakness

General

1. Guillain–Barré syndrome is typically characterized by four phases
   - Prodrome (1–2 weeks)—often following infection, vaccination or surgery
   - Deterioration (1–2 weeks)—progressive motor, sensory and autonomic disturbance
   - Plateau (several days to weeks)—peak paralysis
   - Recovery (several weeks to months)
2. Recovery may be incomplete, particularly in severe cases.
3. Chest infection is a common complication of acute weakness due to inactivity, respiratory and bulbar muscle involvement.

Treatment of Guillain–Barré syndrome

1. Steroids have not shown any benefit in treatment; they may be associated with a higher incidence of relapse.
2. Plasmapheresis or immunoglobulin treatment are useful if used early or in patients requiring mechanical ventilation.
3. Other treatment is supportive including physiotherapy, ventilation as necessary, prevention of pressure sores and muscle contractures etc.

Bibliography

Asbury A, Aranson H, Karp H. Criteria for the diagnosis of Guillain-Barré syndrome. *Ann Neurol* 1978; **3**:565

French Co-operative Group on plasma exchange in Guillain-Barré syndrome. Efficacy of plasma exchange in Guillain-Barré syndrome: role of replacement fluids. *Ann Neurol* 1987; **22**:753

The Guillain–Barré syndrome Study Group. Plasmapheresis and acute Guillain-Barré syndrome. *Neurology* 1985; **35**:1096

Hughes RAC, Newsom-Davies JM, Perkin GD, *et al*. Controlled trial of prednisolone in acute polyneuropathy. *Lancet* 1978; **ii**:750

Hund EF, Borel CO, Cornblath DR, *et al*. Intensive management and treatment of severe Guillain-Barre syndrome. *Crit Care Med* 1993; **21**:433

McLeod JG. Autonomic dysfunction in peripheral nerve disorders. *Curr Opin Neurol Neurosurg* 1992; **5**:476

Ropper AH. The Guillain–Barré syndrome. *N Engl J Med* 1992; **326**:1130

Thomas PK. The Guillain-Barre syndrome: no longer a simple concept. *J Neurol* 1992; **239**:361

Winer J. Guillain-Barre syndrome revisited. *BMJ* 1992; **304**:65

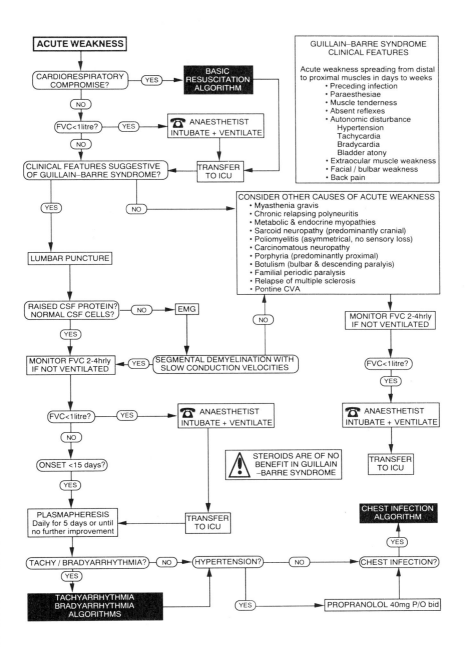

ACUTE WEAKNESS

CARDIORESPIRATORY COMPROMISE? — YES → **BASIC RESUSCITATION ALGORITHM**

NO

FVC<1litre? — YES → ☎ ANAESTHETIST INTUBATE + VENTILATE → TRANSFER TO ICU

NO

CLINICAL FEATURES SUGGESTIVE OF GUILLAIN–BARRE SYNDROME?

GUILLAIN–BARRE SYNDROME
CLINICAL FEATURES

Acute weakness spreading from distal to proximal muscles in days to weeks
• Preceding infection
• Paraesthesiae
• Muscle tenderness
• Absent reflexes
• Autonomic disturbance
   Hypertension
   Tachycardia
   Bradycardia
   Bladder atony
• Extraocular muscle weakness
• Facial / bulbar weakness
• Back pain

YES   NO

CONSIDER OTHER CAUSES OF ACUTE WEAKNESS
• Myasthenia gravis
• Chronic relapsing polyneuritis
• Metabolic & endocrine myopathies
• Sarcoid neuropathy (predominantly cranial)
• Poliomyelitis (asymmetrical, no sensory loss)
• Carcinomatous neuropathy
• Porphyria (predominantly proximal)
• Botulism (bulbar & descending paralyis)
• Familial periodic paralysis
• Relapse of multiple sclerosis
• Pontine CVA

LUMBAR PUNCTURE

RAISED CSF PROTEIN? NORMAL CSF CELLS? — NO → EMG

YES

NO

MONITOR FVC 2-4hrly IF NOT VENTILATED ← YES — SEGMENTAL DEMYELINATION WITH SLOW CONDUCTION VELOCITIES

MONITOR FVC 2-4hrly IF NOT VENTILATED

FVC<1litre? — YES → ☎ ANAESTHETIST INTUBATE + VENTILATE

NO

FVC<1litre?

YES

ONSET <15 days?

⚠ STEROIDS ARE OF NO BENEFIT IN GUILLAIN –BARRE SYNDROME

☎ ANAESTHETIST INTUBATE + VENTILATE

YES

TRANSFER TO ICU

PLASMAPHERESIS Daily for 5 days or until no further improvement ← TRANSFER TO ICU

CHEST INFECTION ALGORITHM

YES

TACHY / BRADYARRHYTHMIA? — NO → HYPERTENSION? — NO → CHEST INFECTION?

YES

TACHYARRHYTHMIA BRADYARRHYTHMIA ALGORITHMS

YES → PROPRANOLOL 40mg P/O bid

8.3 Severe headache and facial pain

Clinical features

1. The history gives the best clues as to the cause of headache:
   - character of pain and whether constant or recurrent
   - duration and time of onset
   - precipitating factors
   - accompanying symptoms
   - age of patient
2. Examination should include assessment of any focal neurological signs, blood pressure, signs of meningeal irritation and areas from which pain may be referred.
3. Although migraine is the commonest cause of severe headache, other more serious causes must be excluded; recurrent, throbbing, often unilateral headache with or without transient neurological deficit suggests migraine.
4. Acute, sudden headache suggests subarachnoid haemorrhage although benign 'thunderclap' headache is recognized.
5. Subacute headache evolving over hours to days may be due to meningitis.
6. Head pain with associated cranial nerve defects may indicate cranial neuralgia; it is often associated with precipitating trigger areas.
7. Temporal arteritis is suggested by temporal headache associated with tenderness over the temporal artery or jaw claudication in the elderly. The full features may not be present. Urgent treatment with steroids is necessary to avoid blindness.

Bibliography

Dechant KL, Clissold SP. Sumatriptan BA. A review of its pharmacodynamic and pharmacokinetic properties, and therapeutic efficacy in the acute treatment of migraine and cluster headache. *Drugs* 1992; **43**:776

Diamond S. Acute headache. Differential diagnosis and management of the three types. *Postgrad Med* 1992; **3**:21

Druce HM. Diagnosis of sinusitis in adults: history, physical examination, nasal cytology, echo, and rhinoscope. *J Allergy Clin Immunol* 1992; **90**:436

Lance JW. Mechanism and management of headache. Butterworths, London, 1982

Silberstein SD. Evaluation and emergency treatment of headache. *Headache* 1992; **32**:396

Ziegler DK. Headache and migraine. *Curr Opin Neurol Neurosurg* 1992; **5**:235

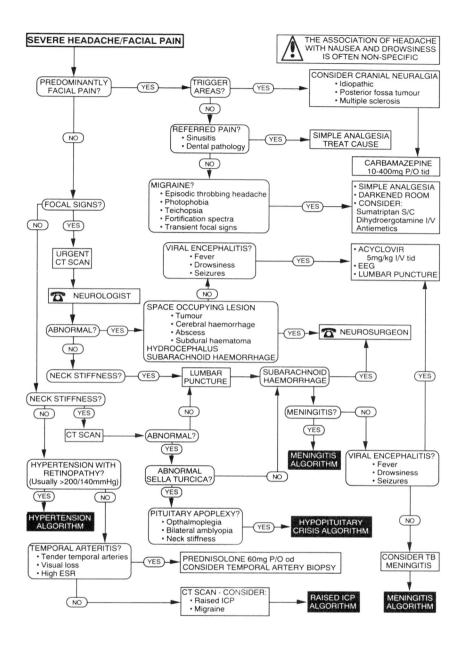

SEVERE HEADACHE/FACIAL PAIN

⚠ THE ASSOCIATION OF HEADACHE WITH NAUSEA AND DROWSINESS IS OFTEN NON-SPECIFIC

PREDOMINANTLY FACIAL PAIN? — YES → TRIGGER AREAS? — YES → CONSIDER CRANIAL NEURALGIA
• Idiopathic
• Posterior fossa tumour
• Multiple sclerosis

NO

REFERRED PAIN?
• Sinusitis
• Dental pathology — YES → SIMPLE ANALGESIA TREAT CAUSE

NO

CARBAMAZEPINE 10-400mg P/O tid

MIGRAINE?
• Episodic throbbing headache
• Photophobia
• Teichopsia
• Fortification spectra
• Transient focal signs — YES →
• SIMPLE ANALGESIA
• DARKENED ROOM
• CONSIDER:
 Sumatriptan S/C
 Dihydroergotamine I/V
 Antiemetics

FOCAL SIGNS?

NO   YES

URGENT CT SCAN

VIRAL ENCEPHALITIS?
• Fever
• Drowsiness
• Seizures — YES →
• ACYCLOVIR 5mg/kg I/V tid
• EEG
• LUMBAR PUNCTURE

☎ NEUROLOGIST

NO

SPACE OCCUPYING LESION
• Tumour
• Cerebral haemorrhage
• Abscess
• Subdural haematoma
HYDROCEPHALUS
SUBARACHNOID HAEMORRHAGE

ABNORMAL? — YES → — YES → ☎ NEUROSURGEON

NO

NECK STIFFNESS? — YES → LUMBAR PUNCTURE → SUBARACHNOID HAEMORRHAGE — YES → — YES →

NECK STIFFNESS?

NO   YES

CT SCAN → ABNORMAL?   NO

MENINGITIS? — NO

YES

YES

HYPERTENSION WITH RETINOPATHY? (Usually >200/140mmHg)

ABNORMAL?

YES

MENINGITIS ALGORITHM

VIRAL ENCEPHALITIS?
• Fever
• Drowsiness
• Seizures

YES   NO

ABNORMAL SELLA TURCICA? — NO

HYPERTENSION ALGORITHM

YES

PITUITARY APOPLEXY?
• Opthalmoplegia
• Bilateral amblyopia
• Neck stiffness — YES → HYPOPITUITARY CRISIS ALGORITHM

NO

TEMPORAL ARTERITIS?
• Tender temporal arteries
• Visual loss
• High ESR — YES → PREDNISOLONE 60mg P/O od CONSIDER TEMPORAL ARTERY BIOPSY

CONSIDER TB MENINGITIS

NO

CT SCAN - CONSIDER:
• Raised ICP
• Migraine → RAISED ICP ALGORITHM

MENINGITIS ALGORITHM

121

8.4 Generalized seizures

1. Control of seizures
   - prevents further hypoxaemic cerebral damage
   - reduces cerebral oxygen requirement
   - reduces raised ICP
2. Always consider underlying disorders such as space-occupying lesions, metabolic disturbances, etc. which require specific treatments.
3. Blood glucose must be checked urgently.
4. Most seizures are self-limiting and require no more than to protect from injury.
5. In known epileptics anticonvulsant levels must be checked. Levels may be inadequate due to poor compliance, concurrent drug therapy or inadequate dosage.

Drug therapy

1. Both benzodiazepines and chlormethiazole may cause respiratory depression and hypoxaemia. The patient *must* be in a well-monitored area if giving a continuous infusion/repeated doses.
2. Phenytoin should not be given intravenously if the patient is taking oral phenytoin and the plasma level is not known.
3. Monitor ECG when giving I/V phenytoin. Give at a rate not exceeding 50 mg/min.
4. If large doses of chlormethiazole are used care should be taken as large volumes of an electrolyte-free solution are being infused.
5. High dose dexamethasone may be used if the patient has a known tumour, arteritis or parasitic CNS infection.
6. In alcoholics thiamine 100 mg I/V should be given.
7. Clonazepam should be used for myoclonic seizures.
8. $MgSO_4$ can be useful for intractable seizures. Loading dose 20 mmol over 20 min. Maintenance dose 10–20 mmol/hr. n.b. maintain good urine output.
9. Sodium valproate can cause severe or fatal liver dysfunction, particularly in combination with other anti-epileptic agents.
10. Phenytoin should not be given orally if patient is on enteral nutrition.

Supportive treatment.

1. Circulation:
   - correct hypoxaemia
   - correct hypovolaemia and electrolyte disturbances (n.b. diabetes insipidus)
2. Generalized seizures may result in hyperthermia which can contribute to cerebral damage.
3. Prevent and treat cerebral oedema:
   - generous sedation
   - hypothermia
   - controlled hyperventilation
   - osmotic diuretics if indicated

Bibliography

Brodie MJ. Status epilepticus in adults. *Lancet* 1990; **336**:551
Fulton B, Park GR. Intravenous chlormethiazole. *Br J Hosp Med* 1992; **48**:742
Jagoda A, Riggio S. Refractory status epilepticus in adults. *Ann Emerg Med* 1993; **22**:1337
Treatment of convulsive status epilepticus. Recommendations of the Epilepsy Foundation of America's Working Group on Status Epilepticus. *JAMA* 1993; **270**:854
Trubuhovich RV. Management of severe or intractable convulsions including eclampsia. *Int Anesthesiol Clin* 1979; **17**:201

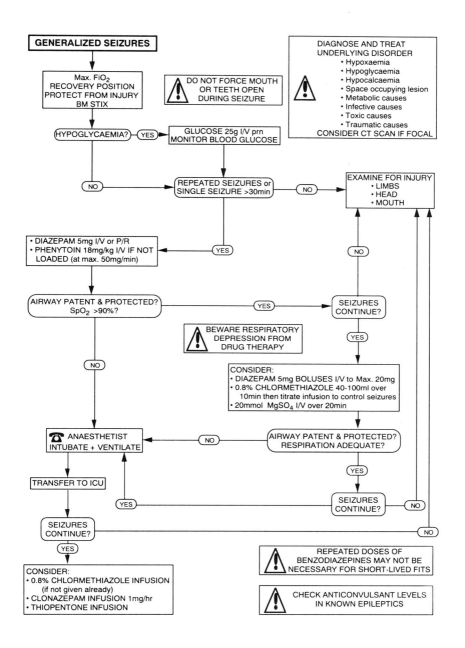

GENERALIZED SEIZURES

Max. FiO$_2$
RECOVERY POSITION
PROTECT FROM INJURY
BM STIX

⚠ DO NOT FORCE MOUTH
OR TEETH OPEN
DURING SEIZURE

DIAGNOSE AND TREAT
UNDERLYING DISORDER
⚠
• Hypoxaemia
• Hypoglycaemia
• Hypocalcaemia
• Space occupying lesion
• Metabolic causes
• Infective causes
• Toxic causes
• Traumatic causes
CONSIDER CT SCAN IF FOCAL

HYPOGLYCAEMIA? ─ YES ─ GLUCOSE 25g I/V prn
MONITOR BLOOD GLUCOSE

NO

REPEATED SEIZURES or
SINGLE SEIZURE >30min ─ NO ─ EXAMINE FOR INJURY
• LIMBS
• HEAD
• MOUTH

• DIAZEPAM 5mg I/V or P/R
• PHENYTOIN 18mg/kg I/V IF NOT
LOADED (at max. 50mg/min) ◄─ YES

AIRWAY PATENT & PROTECTED?
SpO$_2$ >90%? ─── YES ─── SEIZURES
CONTINUE?

⚠ BEWARE RESPIRATORY
DEPRESSION FROM
DRUG THERAPY

NO

YES

CONSIDER:
• DIAZEPAM 5mg BOLUSES I/V to Max. 20mg
• 0.8% CHLORMETHIAZOLE 40-100ml over
10min then titrate infusion to control seizures
• 20mmol MgSO$_4$ I/V over 20min

☎ ANAESTHETIST
INTUBATE + VENTILATE ◄─ NO ─ AIRWAY PATENT & PROTECTED?
RESPIRATION ADEQUATE?

TRANSFER TO ICU

YES

SEIZURES
CONTINUE? ─ YES ─ SEIZURES
CONTINUE? ─ NO

YES

NO

CONSIDER:
• 0.8% CHLORMETHIAZOLE INFUSION
(if not given already)
• CLONAZEPAM INFUSION 1mg/hr
• THIOPENTONE INFUSION

⚠ REPEATED DOSES OF
BENZODIAZEPINES MAY NOT BE
NECESSARY FOR SHORT-LIVED FITS

⚠ CHECK ANTICONVULSANT LEVELS
IN KNOWN EPILEPTICS

8.5 Raised intracranial pressure

General

1. Though intracranial pressure should ideally be kept below 20 mmHg, it is now thought that maintaining cerebral perfusion pressure [CPP] (= mean arterial pressure – intracranial pressure) above 50–60mmHg is more significant.
2. The importance of cerebral blood flow is also now appreciated. The brain may be hyperaemic or hypoxic; reductions in cerebral blood flow (CBF) may be beneficial in the former situation but harmful in the latter. Most of the techniques used to lower ICP also reduce CBF, thereby adding a secondary insult to the primary injury.
3. No bedside non-invasive monitoring technique is generally available to monitor the adequacy of blood flow. Transcranial Doppler ultrasound can measure blood flow in the major cerebral arteries but does not indicate whether or not this supply is adequate. Insertion of a fibreoptic catheter into the jugular venous bulb allows continuous measurement of oxygen saturation. A high value (>75%) indicates hyperaemia whereas a low level (<60%) suggests inadequate flow (provided the arterial oxygen saturation is normal).
4. The jugular venous bulb catheter can also be used for sampling of lactate. A high level suggests inadequate perfusion of the brain.
5. All of these techniques study global changes only; regional areas of cerebral ischaemia may not be identified.

Hyperventilation

1. Hyperventilation (hypocapnia) lowers ICP by cerebral vasoconstriction resulting in a reduction in cerebral blood flow.
2. Hyperventilation to a $PaCO_2$ of 3.5–4.0 has been a mainstay of treatment for raised ICP. However, it is only effective for short periods (4–6 hrs) as the CSF bicarbonate level rapidly adjusts.
3. Hyperventilation may be disadvantageous in low cerebral blood flow states but this will only be recognized by additional monitoring e.g. falling jugular bulb venous O_2 saturation.
4. Rapid increases in $PaCO_2$ should be avoided as this will lead to increases in ICP.
5. Severe alkalosis should be avoided since this increases cerebral vascular resistance and promotes cerebral ischaemia.
6. For acute control of peaks in ICP, further hyperventilation to a $PaCO_2$ of 3.0–3.5 kPa for 10–15 min may be beneficial; however, as in (3) above, it may also be disadvantageous if low flow states are further compromised.

Other therapy

1. Fluid restriction and active diuresis (mannitol and/or frusemide) will usually reduce ICP. This must not be done at the expense of the circulation and cerebral blood flow, especially in low flow states. A plasma osmolality of 310–320 mOsm/kg should not be exceeded.
2. Hyperventilation and fluid restriction will satisfactorily control 80% of cases of raised ICP. Barbiturate therapy will be successful in half of the resistant cases though inotrope/pressor therapy may need to be added. The patient will also require mechanical ventilation.
3. Sedation, analgesia and paralysis will reduce ICP. Coughing, noise, purposeless agitation, excessive physiotherapy and pain should be avoided.
4. Steroids are only useful in raised ICP due to a mass lesion or herpes simplex encephalitis. They have not been shown to be helpful after trauma or ischaemia.

5. Hypertension should not be treated unless very severe. The mean arterial pressure should not usually be reduced below 140–150 mmHg. If treatment is contemplated:
   • Monitor ICP (if possible) to ensure cerebral perfusion pressure is maintained (>50–60 mmHg).
   • Consider the use of β-blockers (if not contraindicated) to decrease the myocardial effects of excessive circulating catecholamines.

Bibliography

Borel C, Hanley D, Diringer MN, Rogers MC. Intensive management of severe head injury. *Chest* 1990; **98**:180

Cruz J. Combined continuous monitoring of systemic and cerebral oxygenation in acute brain injury: Preliminary observations. *Crit Care Med* 1993; **21**: 1225

Cruz J, Raps EC, Hoffstad OJ, Jaggi JL, Gennarelli TA. Cerebral oxygenation monitoring. *Crit Care Med* 1993; **21**: 1242

Dearden NM, Gibson JS, McDowall DG, Gibson RM, Cameron MM. Effect of high-dose dexamethasone on outcome from severe head injury. *J Neurosurg* 1986; **64**:81

Molyneux M, Fox R. Diagnosis and treatment of malaria in Britain. *BMJ* 1993; **306**: 1175

Obrist WD, Langfitt TW, Jaggi JL, Cruz J, Genarelli TA. Cerebral blood flow and metabolism in comatose patients with acute head injury: relationship with intracranial hypertension. *J Neurosurg* 1984; **61**:241

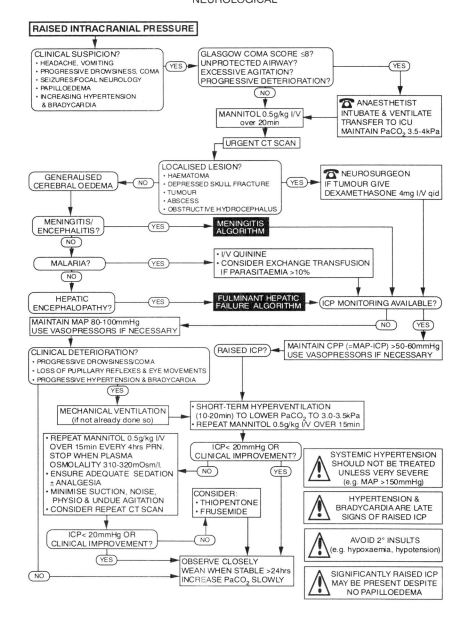

RAISED INTRACRANIAL PRESSURE

CLINICAL SUSPICION?
- HEADACHE, VOMITING
- PROGRESSIVE DROWSINESS, COMA
- SEIZURES/FOCAL NEUROLOGY
- PAPILLOEDEMA
- INCREASING HYPERTENSION & BRADYCARDIA

YES →

GLASGOW COMA SCORE ≤8?
UNPROTECTED AIRWAY?
EXCESSIVE AGITATION?
PROGRESSIVE DETERIORATION?

YES →

NO

☎ ANAESTHETIST
INTUBATE & VENTILATE
TRANSFER TO ICU
MAINTAIN PaCO$_2$ 3.5-4kPa

MANNITOL 0.5g/kg I/V over 20min

URGENT CT SCAN

LOCALISED LESION?
- HAEMATOMA
- DEPRESSED SKULL FRACTURE
- TUMOUR
- ABSCESS
- OBSTRUCTIVE HYDROCEPHALUS

← NO — GENERALISED CEREBRAL OEDEMA

YES → ☎ NEUROSURGEON
IF TUMOUR GIVE
DEXAMETHASONE 4mg I/V qid

MENINGITIS/ENCEPHALITIS?

YES → **MENINGITIS ALGORITHM**

NO

MALARIA?

YES → • I/V QUININE
• CONSIDER EXCHANGE TRANSFUSION IF PARASITAEMIA >10%

NO

HEPATIC ENCEPHALOPATHY?

YES → **FULMINANT HEPATIC FAILURE ALGORITHM**

ICP MONITORING AVAILABLE?

NO   YES

MAINTAIN MAP 80-100mmHg
USE VASOPRESSORS IF NECESSARY

CLINICAL DETERIORATION?
- PROGRESSIVE DROWSINESS/COMA
- LOSS OF PUPILLARY REFLEXES & EYE MOVEMENTS
- PROGRESSIVE HYPERTENSION & BRADYCARDIA

RAISED ICP?

MAINTAIN CPP (=MAP-ICP) >50-60mmHg
USE VASOPRESSORS IF NECESSARY

YES

MECHANICAL VENTILATION
(if not already done so)

• SHORT-TERM HYPERVENTILATION
(10-20min) TO LOWER PaCO$_2$ TO 3.0-3.5kPa
• REPEAT MANNITOL 0.5g/kg I/V OVER 15min

• REPEAT MANNITOL 0.5g/kg I/V OVER 15min EVERY 4hrs PRN. STOP WHEN PLASMA OSMOLALITY 310-320mOsm/l.
• ENSURE ADEQUATE SEDATION ± ANALGESIA
• MINIMISE SUCTION, NOISE, PHYSIO & UNDUE AGITATION
• CONSIDER REPEAT CT SCAN

ICP< 20mmHg OR CLINICAL IMPROVEMENT?

NO   YES

CONSIDER:
• THIOPENTONE
• FRUSEMIDE

NO

ICP< 20mmHg OR CLINICAL IMPROVEMENT?

YES

NO

OBSERVE CLOSELY
WEAN WHEN STABLE >24hrs
INCREASE PaCO$_2$ SLOWLY

⚠ SYSTEMIC HYPERTENSION SHOULD NOT BE TREATED UNLESS VERY SEVERE (e.g. MAP >150mmHg)

⚠ HYPERTENSION & BRADYCARDIA ARE LATE SIGNS OF RAISED ICP

⚠ AVOID 2° INSULTS (e.g. hypoxaemia, hypotension)

⚠ SIGNIFICANTLY RAISED ICP MAY BE PRESENT DESPITE NO PAPILLOEDEMA

Notes

8.6 Acute cerebrovascular accident

General

1. A stroke usually produces an acute neurological deterioration occurring over seconds to hours
2. Transient episodes may precede the event and are often embolic in origin from carotid or cardiac sources.
3. A cardiac embolic cause is more likely with longstanding arrhythmias, haemorrhage or thrombosis with hypertension, and thromboembolism in longstanding smokers or diabetics. Vasculitis should be considered in patients with connective tissue disorders.
4. Risk factors for CVA include hypertension, smoking, diabetes, atrial fibrillation, polycythaemia, contraceptive steroids, obesity, hyperlipidaemia, hyperfibrinogenaemia.
5. An urgent CT scan should be considered if a CVA occurs in a patient <50 years old, in an atypical presentation (e.g. post-trauma), if a haemorrhagic cause needs to be excluded (e.g. to commence anticoagulation), or if it affects the brain stem or cerebellar areas (e.g. quadriplegia, disturbances of gaze or vision, locked-in syndrome). The regional neurosurgical centre should be contacted.
6. An echocardiogram should be performed if an embolic cause is suspected. Endocarditis should be considered.
7. The risk of a stroke following TIA is 5% per annum.
8. Temporal arteritis may present with tender temporal arteries, sudden blindness or a stroke affecting the vertebral territory. The ESR is elevated. Steroids should be started promptly before the results of temporal artery biopsy are known.
9. Prevention of secondary insults, e.g. hypoxaemia, hypotension, is crucial.

Treatment

1. Hypertension should not be generally treated at the outset unless very high e.g. mean arterial pressure above 140 mmHg, or a diastolic pressure above 120 mmHg. If treatment is necessary, the MAP should not be lowered below 130 mmHg or the diastolic below 110 mmHg in the first 48 hours.
2. Aspirin or warfarin should be given for embolic causes unless contraindicated. Similarly, thrombolytics such as streptokinase should be considered at an early stage (within 6 hours) provided cerebral haemorrhage is excluded and there are no other contraindications.
3. If a supraventricular arrhythmia is present, the rate should be controlled and the patient anticoagulated provided cerebral haemorrhage is excluded and there are no other contraindications.

Subarachnoid haemorrhage

1. In 15% of cases no cause is found. Otherwise, 80% are due to ruptured aneurysm, 5% to arteriovenous malformations and 15% to trauma.
2. The patient may present with neck stiffness, cranial nerve palsies, drowsiness ± hemiplegia, and prolonged coma.
3. Diagnosis is by CT scan or by lumbar puncture revealing xanthochromia or bloody CSF not clearing by the third sample.
4. Patients surviving 1 month have a 90% chance of surviving 1 year.
5. Rebleeding occurs in 30%.
6. The optimal time for surgical intervention is controversial. Local policies will differ thus the neurosurgical centre should always be consulted.
7. Nimodipine has been shown to improve outcome.

ACUTE CEREBROVASCULAR ACCIDENT

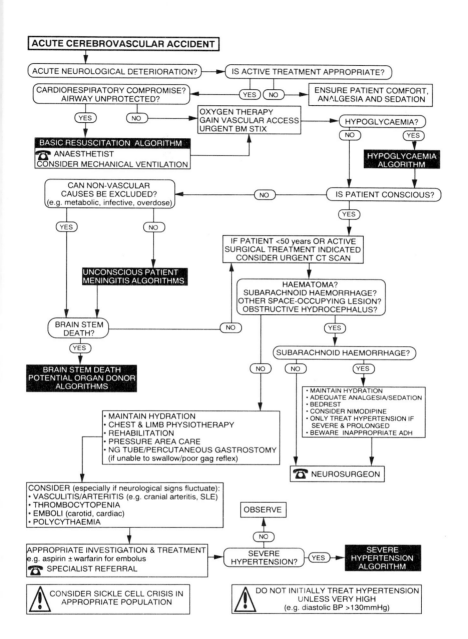

ACUTE NEUROLOGICAL DETERIORATION? → IS ACTIVE TREATMENT APPROPRIATE?

CARDIORESPIRATORY COMPROMISE? AIRWAY UNPROTECTED?

YES / NO

ENSURE PATIENT COMFORT, ANALGESIA AND SEDATION

YES / NO

OXYGEN THERAPY
GAIN VASCULAR ACCESS
URGENT BM STIX

HYPOGLYCAEMIA?

NO / YES

BASIC RESUSCITATION ALGORITHM
☎ ANAESTHETIST
CONSIDER MECHANICAL VENTILATION

HYPOGLYCAEMIA ALGORITHM

CAN NON-VASCULAR CAUSES BE EXCLUDED?
(e.g. metabolic, infective, overdose)

NO ← IS PATIENT CONSCIOUS?

YES / NO

YES

IF PATIENT <50 years OR ACTIVE SURGICAL TREATMENT INDICATED CONSIDER URGENT CT SCAN

UNCONSCIOUS PATIENT MENINGITIS ALGORITHMS

HAEMATOMA?
SUBARACHNOID HAEMORRHAGE?
OTHER SPACE-OCCUPYING LESION?
OBSTRUCTIVE HYDROCEPHALUS?

BRAIN STEM DEATH? — NO

YES

SUBARACHNOID HAEMORRHAGE?

BRAIN STEM DEATH POTENTIAL ORGAN DONOR ALGORITHMS

NO / NO / YES

• MAINTAIN HYDRATION
• ADEQUATE ANALGESIA/SEDATION
• BEDREST
• CONSIDER NIMODIPINE
• ONLY TREAT HYPERTENSION IF SEVERE & PROLONGED
• BEWARE INAPPROPRIATE ADH

• MAINTAIN HYDRATION
• CHEST & LIMB PHYSIOTHERAPY
• REHABILITATION
• PRESSURE AREA CARE
• NG TUBE/PERCUTANEOUS GASTROSTOMY
(if unable to swallow/poor gag reflex)

☎ NEUROSURGEON

CONSIDER (especially if neurological signs fluctuate):
• VASCULITIS/ARTERITIS (e.g. cranial arteritis, SLE)
• THROMBOCYTOPENIA
• EMBOLI (carotid, cardiac)
• POLYCYTHAEMIA

OBSERVE

NO

APPROPRIATE INVESTIGATION & TREATMENT
e.g. aspirin ± warfarin for embolus
☎ SPECIALIST REFERRAL

SEVERE HYPERTENSION? — YES

SEVERE HYPERTENSION ALGORITHM

⚠ CONSIDER SICKLE CELL CRISIS IN APPROPRIATE POPULATION

⚠ DO NOT INITIALLY TREAT HYPERTENSION UNLESS VERY HIGH
(e.g. diastolic BP >130mmHg)

Bibliography

Bayer AJ, Pathy MS, Newcombe R. Double-blind randomised trial of intravenous glycerol in acute stroke., *Lancet* 1987; **i**: 405

Grotta JC. Current medical and surgical therapy for cerebrovascular disease. *N Engl J Med* 1987; **317**: 1505

Pickard JD, Murray GD, Illingworth R. *et al.* Effect of oral nimodipine on cerebral infarction and outcome after subarachnoid haemorrhage: British aneurysm nimodipine trial. *BMJ* 1989; **298**: 636

Sandercock P, Molyneux A, Warlow C. Value of computed tomography in patients with stroke: Oxfordshire Community Stroke Project. *BMJ* 1985; **290**: 193

Sandercock P. Important new treatments for acute ischaemic stroke. *BMJ* 1987; **295**: 1224

Notes

8.7 Meningitis

General
1. Meningitis is a life-threatening but potentially salvageable condition that requires prompt action.
2. A low threshold of suspicion for meningitis should be harboured in any patient presenting with an alteration in conscious level.
3. Signs of meningism need not necessarily be present.

Lumbar puncture
1. In view of the risk of coning if intracranial pressure is elevated, it is safer to start antibiotics presumptively at the earliest opportunity. A lumbar puncture (LP) should only be performed if one is confident that ICP is not elevated, if doubt remains or focal signs are present, after CT exclusion.
   n.b. a CT scan does not necessarily exclude raised ICP.
2. If considerable delay is envisaged before a LP is performed, antibiotics should be commenced empirically on 'best guess' diagnosis (see below).
3. Typical CSF values

	Pyogenic	Viral	TB
appearance	turbid	clear	fibrin web
predominant cell type	polymorphs	lymphocytes	lymphocytes
cell count/mm^3	>1000	<500	50–1500
protein (g/litre)	>1	0.5–1	1–5
CSF:blood glucose	<60%	>60%	<60%

4. Rarer causes of meningitis include TB, leptospirosis and brucellosis; the CSF reveals no organisms but a high lymphocyte count is present.
5. If indicated, send CSF for acid fast stain (TB) and India Ink stain (Cryptococcus).
6. An early LP may be normal in pyogenic meningitis. If necessary, repeat LP.

Treatment

Organism	Patients commonly affected	Antibiotic and dosage regimen (alternatives in brackets)
Pneumococcus	older adults	benzylpenicillin 1.2 g I/V 2–4hrly (chloramphenicol 12.5 mg/kg I/V 6 hrly)
Meningococcus	young adults	benzyl penicillin 1.2 g I/V 2–4 hrly (chloramphenicol 12.5 mg/kg I/V 6 hrly)
Haemophilus influenzae	young children	chloramphenicol 12.5 mg/kg I/V 6 hrly (cefotaxime 50 mg/kg I/V 8 hrly)
Listeria monocytogenes	elderly, immunocompromised	ampicillin 1 g I/V 4–6hrly + gentamicin 120 mg I/V stat, then 80 mg 8–12 hrly (given according to plasma levels)
Mycobacterium tuberculosis	elderly, immunocompromised	quadruple therapy (rifampicin/isoniazid/ ethambutol/pyrazinamide)
Cryptococcus neoformans	immunocompromised	amphotericin B starting at 250 µg/kg I/V od + flucytosine 50 mg/kg I/V 6 hrly
Staph. aureus	immunocompromised	flucloxacillin 2 g I/V 6 hrly
E.coli	neonates, immunocompromised	cefotaxime 50 mg/kg I/V od

1. Change antibiotic if necessary once organism and sensitivities known.
2. Continue parenteral antibiotics for minimum of 10 days.

3. Dexamethasone has been shown to reduce the incidence of complications and improve the outcome in bacterial meningitis in children.
4. Rifampicin should be given to all family and close social contacts of meningococcal (600 mg P/O 12 hrly for 2 days) and haemophilus (600 mg P/O od for 4 days) meningitis. The index case should also receive these doses before discharge home.

Aseptic meningitis
1. Causes include:
   • viruses (echo, mumps, measles, etc.)
   • Lyme disease
   • leptospirosis, listeriosis, brucellosis
   • fungi
   • atypical TB
   • sarcoidosis, SLE
   • partially treated bacterial meningitis

Bibliography
Archer BD. Computed tomography before lumbar puncture in acute meningitis: a review of the risks and benefits. *Can Med Assoc J* 1993; **148**: 961
Talan DA, Zibulewsky J. Relationship of clinical presentation to time of antibiotics for the emergency department management of suspected bacterial meningitis. *Ann Emerg Med* 1993; **22**: 1733
Thompson J. Role of glucocorticoids in the treatment of infectious diseases. *Eur J Clin Microbiol Infect Dis* **12** (Suppl.1) S68

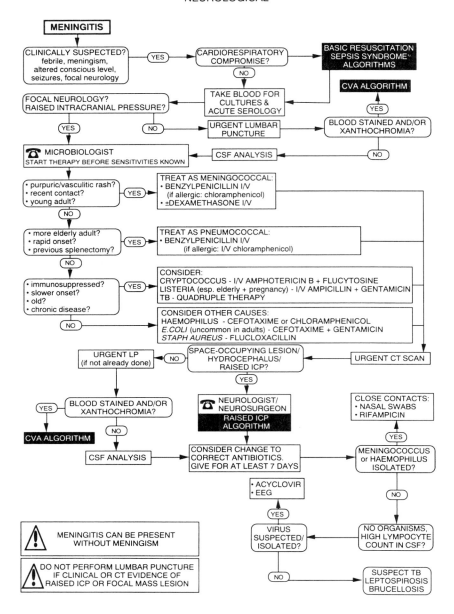

Notes

8.8 Severe myasthenia

General
1. Myasthenia gravis is associated with other autoimmune diseases such as thyroid disease, SLE, rheumatoid arthritis. Autoantibody screens should include investigation of these diseases as well as antibodies specific to myasthenia gravis.
2. Tendon reflexes are spared and weakness is painless in myasthenia unlike some of the alternative causes of weakness.
3. The myasthenic-myopathic syndrome associated with carcinoma of the bronchus may respond to the edrophonium (Tensilon) test but there is not a sustained response to anticholinesterase treatment.
4. Anticholinesterase treatment is symptomatic; steroids and azathioprine give the best chance of pharmacological remission.
5. In patients with a thymoma or patients <45 years old (usually females) thymectomy gives the best chance of remission.

The edrophonium (Tensilon) test
1. Edrophonium is a short acting anticholinesterase.
2. If no cholinergic side-effects (sweating, salivation, lacrimation, colic, fasiculation etc.) are seen after 2 mg I/V a further 8 mg may be given to assess response.
3. Atropine (1 mg I/V) should be available to combat cholinergic side-effects and may be given prophylactically.
4. A positive test is judged by improvement in weakness of muscle groups most severely affected occuring within 3 minutes of injection.
5. The test can be combined with objective assessment of respiratory function by monitoring FVC response or by assessing the response to repetitive stimulation with an EMG.
6. When attempting to distinguish between a myasthenic and a cholinergic crisis an anaesthetist should be immediately available to intubate and ventilate the patient as necessary.

Myasthenic crisis
1. Usually occurs in known myasthenics during stress, infection, trauma or childbirth but may be the presenting feature.
2. Early treatment of myasthenia with steroids may cause a deterioration for up to 2 weeks.
3. Myasthenic crisis may be difficult to distinguish from cholinergic crisis.
4. Some patients may experience improvement in some muscle groups with pyridostigmine but a cholinergic crisis affecting others due to differential sensitivity.
5. If myasthenic crisis fails to respond to increased doses of pyridostigmine all drugs should be stopped and respiration supported as necessary; this should allow distinction from cholinergic crisis.
6. In severe myasthenic crisis plasmapheresis to remove the autoantibody load may be life saving.

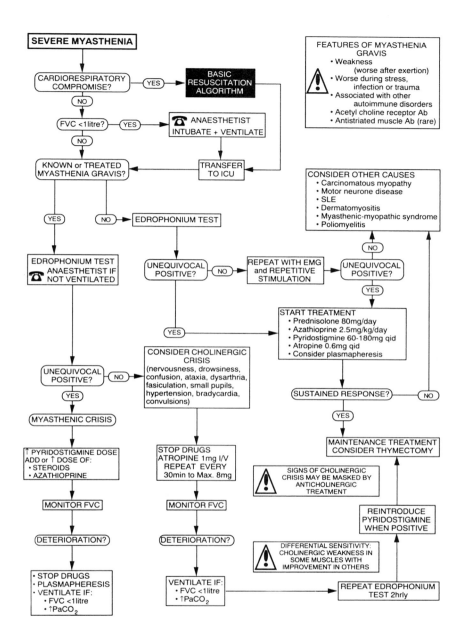

SEVERE MYASTHENIA

CARDIORESPIRATORY COMPROMISE? — YES → **BASIC RESUSCITATION ALGORITHM**

NO

FVC <1litre? — YES → ☎ ANAESTHETIST INTUBATE + VENTILATE

NO

KNOWN or TREATED MYASTHENIA GRAVIS? ← TRANSFER TO ICU

YES | NO → EDROPHONIUM TEST

EDROPHONIUM TEST ☎ ANAESTHETIST IF NOT VENTILATED

UNEQUIVOCAL POSITIVE? — NO → REPEAT WITH EMG and REPETITIVE STIMULATION → UNEQUIVOCAL POSITIVE?

YES

YES

FEATURES OF MYASTHENIA GRAVIS
⚠
• Weakness (worse after exertion)
• Worse during stress, infection or trauma
• Associated with other autoimmune disorders
• Acetyl choline receptor Ab
• Antistriated muscle Ab (rare)

CONSIDER OTHER CAUSES
• Carcinomatous myopathy
• Motor neurone disease
• SLE
• Dermatomyositis
• Myasthenic-myopathic syndrome
• Poliomyelitis

NO

START TREATMENT
• Prednisolone 80mg/day
• Azathioprine 2.5mg/kg/day
• Pyridostigmine 60-180mg qid
• Atropine 0.6mg qid
• Consider plasmapheresis

CONSIDER CHOLINERGIC CRISIS
(nervousness, drowsiness, confusion, ataxia, dysarthria, fasiculation, small pupils, hypertension, bradycardia, convulsions)

UNEQUIVOCAL POSITIVE? — NO

YES

MYASTHENIC CRISIS

SUSTAINED RESPONSE? — NO

YES

MAINTENANCE TREATMENT CONSIDER THYMECTOMY

↑ PYRIDOSTIGMINE DOSE ADD or ↑ DOSE OF:
• STEROIDS
• AZATHIOPRINE

STOP DRUGS ATROPINE 1mg I/V REPEAT EVERY 30min to Max. 8mg

⚠ SIGNS OF CHOLINERGIC CRISIS MAY BE MASKED BY ANTICHOLINERGIC TREATMENT

MONITOR FVC

MONITOR FVC

REINTRODUCE PYRIDOSTIGMINE WHEN POSITIVE

DETERIORATION?

DETERIORATION?

⚠ DIFFERENTIAL SENSITIVITY: CHOLINERGIC WEAKNESS IN SOME MUSCLES WITH IMPROVEMENT IN OTHERS

• STOP DRUGS
• PLASMAPHERESIS
• VENTILATE IF:
  • FVC <1litre
  • ↑PaCO$_2$

VENTILATE IF:
• FVC <1litre
• ↑PaCO$_2$

REPEAT EDROPHONIUM TEST 2hrly

Cholinergic crisis

1. Symptoms are worst within 2 hr of last dose of anticholinesterase. Many clinical features may be masked by concurrent treatment with anticholinergics.
2. Atropine is the mainstay of treatment after stopping anticholinesterases and supporting respiration as necessary.
3. Repeated edrophonium tests 2 hrly allow assessment of reformation of plasma cholinesterases after which pyridostigmine can be reintroduced.

Bibliography

Drachman DB, McIntosh KR, Reim J, *et al.* Strategies for treatment of myasthenia gravis. *Ann N Y Acad Sci* 1993; **681**:515

Newsom-Davis J, Vincent A. Myasthenia gravis. In: Lachmann PJ, Peters DK (Eds) Clinical aspects of immunology. Blackwell Scientific, Oxford,1982, p1011

Oosterhuis HJ, Kuks JB. Myasthenia gravis and myasthenic syndromes. *Curr Opin Neurol Neurosurg* 1992; **5**:638

Scadding GK, Harvard GWH. Pathogenesis and treatment of myasthenia gravis. *BMJ* 1981; **2**:1008

Notes

8.9 Tetanus

General

1. Tetanus is the clinical syndrome caused by the exotoxin, tetanospasmin, from the anaerobe *Clostridium tetani* in contaminated and devitalized wounds.
2. Tetanus toxin ascends intra-axonally in motor and autonomic nerves blocking release of inhibitory neurotransmitters.
3. The incubation period between contamination and onset is of variable length; shorter incubation periods imply a larger toxin load and therefore very severe disease.
4. Previous active immunization may modify the disease such that milder symptoms are seen with larger toxin loads or spasms are localized to muscles close to the site of injury.

Treatment

1. The disease is self-limiting; treatment is therefore supportive and to prevent complications. Passive immunization may shorten the course of the disease by removing the circulating toxin load but rapid fixation of toxin to tissues limits the usefulness of this approach.
2. Surgical debridement of the wound and antibiotic therapy is of paramount importance to remove the source of the toxin.
3. Muscle spasms are provoked by stimulation; a quiet environment with minimum disturbance and sedation help prevent spasms.
4. Treatment of muscle spasms requires a benzodiazepine and/or chlorpromazine.
5. Asphyxia due to prolonged and severe respiratory muscle spasm or laryngospasm can be prevented by sedation and muscle relaxation.
6. Autonomic complications are best prevented by deep sedation or anaesthesia supplemented as necessary by autonomic blockade. Magnesium may also prevent sympathetic overactivity.
7. All patients must be actively immunized before discharge since the disease confers no immunity.

Bibliography

Dolar D. The use of continuous atropine infusion in the management of severe tetanus. *Intensive Care Med* 1992; **18**:26

James MFM, Manson EDB. The use of magnesium sulphate infusions in the management of very severe tetanus. *Intensive Care Med* 1985; **11**:5

Prys-Roberts C, Kerr JH, Corbett JL, *et al.* Treatment of sympathetic overactivity in tetanus. *Lancet* 1969; **i**:542

Smith JWG, Laurence DR, Evans DG. Prevention of tetanus in the wounded. *Br Med J* 1975; **iii**:453

Trujillo MH, Castillo A, Espana JV, *et al.* Tetanus in the adult: Intensive care and management experience with 233 cases. *Crit Care Med* 1980; **7**:419

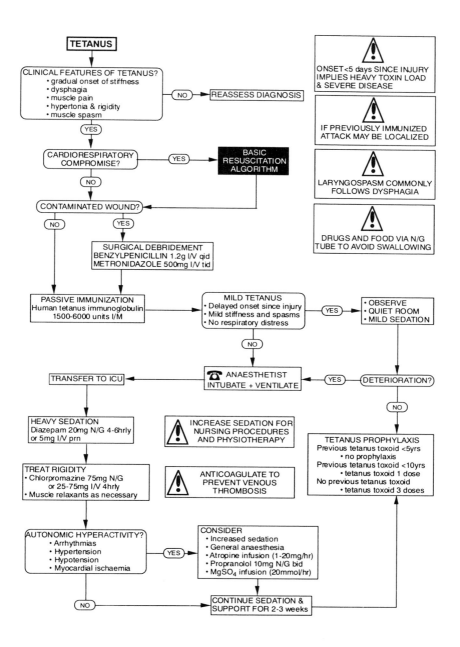

TETANUS

CLINICAL FEATURES OF TETANUS?
- gradual onset of stiffness
- dysphagia
- muscle pain
- hypertonia & rigidity
- muscle spasm

NO → REASSESS DIAGNOSIS

YES

CARDIORESPIRATORY COMPROMISE? — YES → **BASIC RESUSCITATION ALGORITHM**

NO

CONTAMINATED WOUND?

NO   YES

SURGICAL DEBRIDEMENT
BENZYLPENICILLIN 1.2g I/V qid
METRONIDAZOLE 500mg I/V tid

PASSIVE IMMUNIZATION
Human tetanus immunoglobulin
1500-6000 units I/M

MILD TETANUS
- Delayed onset since injury
- Mild stiffness and spasms
- No respiratory distress

YES →
- OBSERVE
- QUIET ROOM
- MILD SEDATION

NO

TRANSFER TO ICU ← ☎ ANAESTHETIST INTUBATE + VENTILATE ← YES — DETERIORATION?

NO

HEAVY SEDATION
Diazepam 20mg N/G 4-6hrly
or 5mg I/V prn

⚠ INCREASE SEDATION FOR NURSING PROCEDURES AND PHYSIOTHERAPY

TREAT RIGIDITY
- Chlorpromazine 75mg N/G or 25-75mg I/V 4hrly
- Muscle relaxants as necessary

⚠ ANTICOAGULATE TO PREVENT VENOUS THROMBOSIS

TETANUS PROPHYLAXIS
Previous tetanus toxoid <5yrs
- no prophylaxis
Previous tetanus toxoid <10yrs
- tetanus toxoid 1 dose
No previous tetanus toxoid
- tetanus toxoid 3 doses

AUTONOMIC HYPERACTIVITY?
- Arrhythmias
- Hypertension
- Hypotension
- Myocardial ischaemia

YES →
CONSIDER
- Increased sedation
- General anaesthesia
- Atropine infusion (1-20mg/hr)
- Propranolol 10mg N/G bid
- MgSO$_4$ infusion (20mmol/hr)

NO →

CONTINUE SEDATION & SUPPORT FOR 2-3 weeks

⚠ ONSET <5 days SINCE INJURY IMPLIES HEAVY TOXIN LOAD & SEVERE DISEASE

⚠ IF PREVIOUSLY IMMUNIZED ATTACK MAY BE LOCALIZED

⚠ LARYNGOSPASM COMMONLY FOLLOWS DYSPHAGIA

⚠ DRUGS AND FOOD VIA N/G TUBE TO AVOID SWALLOWING

8.10 Brain stem death

1. Brain stem death is usually followed by asystole within a few days.
2. The correct diagnosis of brain stem death is a form of medical emergency in that it allows:
   - discontinuation of pointless mechanical ventilation
   - retrieval of organs for donation
3. A checklist of brainstem death tests and a special chart to record tests is useful.
4. It is essential to have a diagnosis of a disorder which may cause brain stem death.
5. Drugs or metabolic disturbances which may depress the brain must be excluded before brain stem death can be pronounced.
6. An initially negative brain stem death test may, on repetition, hours or days later, become positive. The converse, however, cannot happen.
7. Discussion of brain stem death tests and (if indicated) organ donation must include the family and all medical and nursing staff who are involved.
8. A member of the transplant team should not ideally perform brain stem death testing.

Bibliography

Cadaveric organs for transplantation. A code of practice including the diagnosis of brain death. Department of Health, London, 1983
Jennett B. Brain death. *Br J Anaesth* 1981; **53**: 1111

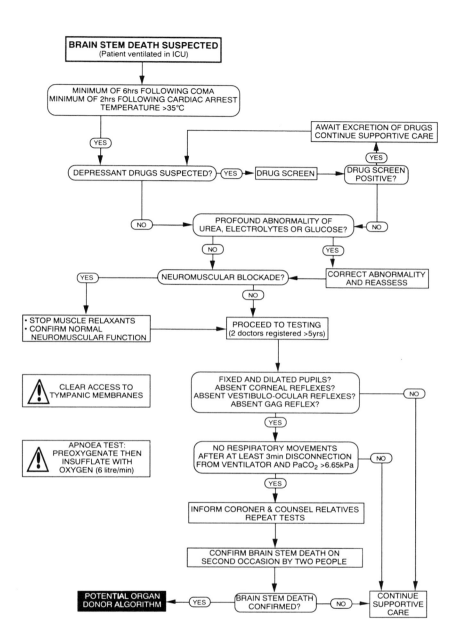

BRAIN STEM DEATH SUSPECTED
(Patient ventilated in ICU)

MINIMUM OF 6hrs FOLLOWING COMA
MINIMUM OF 2hrs FOLLOWING CARDIAC ARREST
TEMPERATURE >35°C

YES

AWAIT EXCRETION OF DRUGS
CONTINUE SUPPORTIVE CARE

YES

DEPRESSANT DRUGS SUSPECTED? — YES → DRUG SCREEN → DRUG SCREEN POSITIVE?

NO

NO

PROFOUND ABNORMALITY OF
UREA, ELECTROLYTES OR GLUCOSE?

NO

YES

YES

NEUROMUSCULAR BLOCKADE? ← CORRECT ABNORMALITY AND REASSESS

NO

• STOP MUSCLE RELAXANTS
• CONFIRM NORMAL
NEUROMUSCULAR FUNCTION

PROCEED TO TESTING
(2 doctors registered >5yrs)

⚠ CLEAR ACCESS TO TYMPANIC MEMBRANES

FIXED AND DILATED PUPILS?
ABSENT CORNEAL REFLEXES?
ABSENT VESTIBULO-OCULAR REFLEXES?
ABSENT GAG REFLEX?

NO

YES

⚠ APNOEA TEST:
PREOXYGENATE THEN
INSUFFLATE WITH
OXYGEN (6 litre/min)

NO RESPIRATORY MOVEMENTS
AFTER AT LEAST 3min DISCONNECTION
FROM VENTILATOR AND PaCO$_2$ >6.65kPa

NO

YES

INFORM CORONER & COUNSEL RELATIVES
REPEAT TESTS

CONFIRM BRAIN STEM DEATH ON
SECOND OCCASION BY TWO PEOPLE

POTENTIAL ORGAN
DONOR ALGORITHM ← YES — BRAIN STEM DEATH CONFIRMED? — NO → CONTINUE SUPPORTIVE CARE

8.11 Potential organ donor

1. Treatment of many patients with chronic renal failure, cardiac failure, hepatic failure and some forms of chronic respiratory failure is critically dependent on organ donation. Organ donors mainly come from the ICU.
2. Always consider the possibility of the patient becoming an organ donor which, in itself, may be a reason for admission to the ICU.
3. Consult the local transplant coordinator early.
4. Suitability of organs for donation must be confirmed with the transplant coordinator; as a guide:
   - Kidneys—Age 4–70, acceptable U & E and creatinine
   - Heart—Age 0–50, acceptable CXR and ECG
   - Lungs—Age 0–50, acceptable CXR and blood gases
   - Liver—Age 0–55, no alcohol or drug abuse, acceptable LFTs
   - Corneas—Age 0–100, no previous intraocular surgery
5. Do not reject brain dead potential donors e.g. with fully treated infections or acute renal failure without consultation with the transplant coordinator.
6. Maintain organs of brain stem dead patients in optimal condition for transplantation, e.g. avoid hypotension, fluid imbalance, etc.

Bibliography

Gore SM, Hinds CJ, Rutherford AJ. Organ donation from intensive care units in England. *BMJ* 1989; **249**: 1193

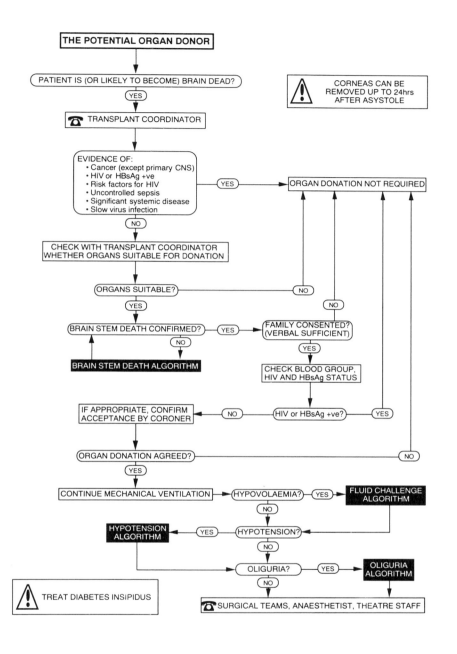

THE POTENTIAL ORGAN DONOR

PATIENT IS (OR LIKELY TO BECOME) BRAIN DEAD?
YES

☎ TRANSPLANT COORDINATOR

CORNEAS CAN BE
REMOVED UP TO 24hrs
AFTER ASYSTOLE

EVIDENCE OF:
• Cancer (except primary CNS)
• HiV or HBsAg +ve
• Risk factors for HIV
• Uncontrolled sepsis
• Significant systemic disease
• Slow virus infection
YES → ORGAN DONATION NOT REQUIRED
NO

CHECK WITH TRANSPLANT COORDINATOR
WHETHER ORGANS SUITABLE FOR DONATION

ORGANS SUITABLE? — NO
YES
NO

BRAIN STEM DEATH CONFIRMED? — YES → FAMILY CONSENTED?
(VERBAL SUFFICIENT)
NO
YES

BRAIN STEM DEATH ALGORITHM

CHECK BLOOD GROUP,
HIV AND HBsAg STATUS

IF APPROPRIATE, CONFIRM
ACCEPTANCE BY CORONER ← NO — HIV or HBsAg +ve? — YES

ORGAN DONATION AGREED? — NO
YES

CONTINUE MECHANICAL VENTILATION → HYPOVOLAEMIA? — YES → **FLUID CHALLENGE ALGORITHM**
NO

HYPOTENSION ALGORITHM ← YES — HYPOTENSION?
NO

OLIGURIA? — YES → **OLIGURIA ALGORITHM**
NO

⚠ TREAT DIABETES INSIPIDUS

☎ SURGICAL TEAMS, ANAESTHETIST, THEATRE STAFF

145

9. Poisoning

9.1 Acute poisoning

Diagnosis
1. Usually the history is obvious. Physical signs may be absent or confused due to ingestion of mixed poisons.
2. Urgent advice should be sought from a poisons information centre.
3. Some poisons may cause toxicity without ingestion, e.g. by inhalation or through the skin.
4. Blood levels of salicylate and paracetamol are required in all cases of poisoning since active treatment will be required. A qualitative drug screen is a useful aid to diagnosis.
5. In some cases the effects of poisoning are late (e.g. paracetamol, paraquat).

Elimination of poisons from the stomach
1. Ipecacuanha-induced vomiting may be delayed for up to 30 min and then may be intractable.
2. No clear advantages have been documented for either ipecacuanha or gastric lavage.
3. Aspiration is a serious risk with any form of gastric emptying therapy; the patient should be intubated for airway protection if consciousness is at all obtunded.
4. Gastric emptying should not be used if corrosives or hydrocarbons have been ingested; in these cases give milk orally.
5. Activated charcoal is probably more effective than gastric emptying procedures to prevent drug absorption but requires a charcoal:poison weight ratio of 10:1.
6. Elimination of drugs from the circulation may be achieved via the small bowel by repeated doses of activated charcoal; a dose of 50–100 g is given initially followed by 12.5 g/hr via a N/G tube.

Other elimination techniques
1. For most patients supportive therapy will suffice. However, for severe poisoning forced diuresis with appropriate urinary acidification or alkalinization, or haemodialysis may be useful.
2. These techniques are only useful for poisons that are water soluble and distributed predominantly extracellularly.
3. A forced diuresis of >200 ml/hr should be maintained with frusemide or mannitol, in addition to intravenous crystalloids (500 ml 5% glucose alternating with 500 ml 0.9% saline).
4. The volume of crystalloid infused should be sufficient to prevent hypovolaemia but care should be taken to avoid an excessively positive fluid balance.
5. Forced diuresis techniques should be abandoned if renal function is abnormal.
6. During a forced alkaline diuresis urinary pH should be maintained between 7.5 and 8.5 with 1.26% sodium bicarbonate solution (to replace the 0.9% saline). Arterial pH should not be allowed to increase above 7.5. Bicarbonate infusion should be stopped if the arterial pH is high.
7. Increased urinary alkali excretion is associated with hypokalaemia; careful monitoring and replacement of potassium is necessary.
8. If urine fails to alkalinize with bicarbonate infusion further potassium repletion will be required.

9. During a forced acid diuresis urinary pH should be maintained below 7.0 by adding 750 mg ammonium chloride to each 500 ml 5% glucose alternating with 500 ml 0.9% saline.

Antidotes

1. Few specific antidotes to poisons are available:

Poison	Antidote
Anticholinergics	Physostigmine
Benzodiazepines	Flumazenil
Digoxin	Fab digoxin specific antibody
Ethylene glycol	Ethanol
Iron	Desferrioxamine
Methanol	Ethanol
Opiates	Naloxone
Organophosphorus compounds	Pralidoxime + atropine
Paracetamol	N-acetylcysteine

2. Naloxone and flumazenil should be used with caution since ventricular fibrillation and seizures may be precipitated.

Bibliography

Kulig K. Initial management of ingestins of toxic substances. *N Engl J Med* 1992; **326**:1677

Neuvonen PJ, Vartiainen M, Tokola O. Comparison of activated charcoal and ipecac syrup in prevention of drug absorption. *Eur J Clin Pharmacol* 1983; **24**:557

Tandberg D, Diven BG, McLeod JM. Ipecac induced emesis versus gastric lavage: a controlled study in normal adults. *Am J Emerg Med* 1986; **4**:205

Wenger TL, Butler VP, Habet E, *et al.* Treatment of 63 severely digitalis-toxic patients with digoxin-specific antibody fragments. *J Am Coll Cardiol* 1985; **5**:118A

Young MF, Bivins HG. Evaluation of gastric emptying using radionuclides: gastric lavage versus ipecac-induced emesis. *Ann Emerg Med* 1991; **20**:952

POISONING

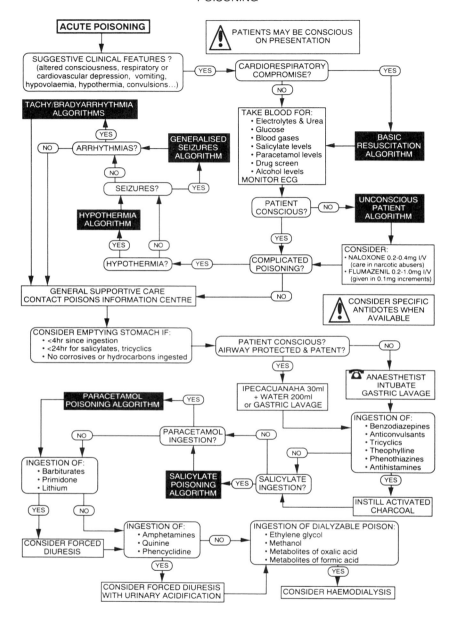

Notes

9.2 Paracetamol poisoning

Toxicity of paracetamol
1. Serious, life-threatening toxicity is likely after ingestion of >15 g paracetamol.
2. Paracetamol is rapidly absorbed from the stomach and upper small bowel. It is metabolized by conjugation in the liver.
3. Hepatic necrosis is due to an alkylating metabolite of paracetamol which is normally removed by conjugation with glutathione but this is rapidly depleted with overdose.
4. Hepatic toxicity is usually asymptomatic for 1–2 days. Laboratory tests may start to become abnormal after 18 hr but, more commonly, abnormalities are seen at 3–5 days.
5. Hepatic failure, if manifest, develops at 2–7 days, a more severe overdose being associated with a more rapid onset of hepatic failure.

Prevention of paracetamol-induced liver damage
1. Early restoration of hepatic glutathione levels with its precursor, N-acetylcysteine, is the mainstay of treatment.
2. N-acetylcysteine is most effective if started within 10 hr of ingestion but can be useful up to 36 hr after ingestion.

Referral to specialist centre
1. Referral should be early since patients with established hepatic failure do not travel well.
2. A rise in prothrombin time or bilirubin is an early warning of significant hepatic damage.

Bibliography
Harrison PM, Keays R, Bray GP, *et al*. Improved outcome of paracetamol induced fulminant hepatic failure by late administration of acetylcysteine. *Lancet* 1990; **i**:1572
Prescott LF. Treatment of severe acetaminophen poisoning with intravenous acetylcysteine. *Arch Intern Med* 1981; **141**:386

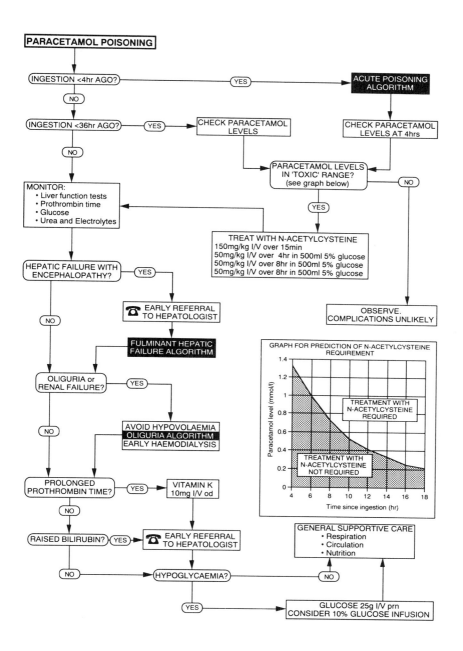

PARACETAMOL POISONING

INGESTION <4hr AGO? —YES→ **ACUTE POISONING ALGORITHM**

NO ↓

INGESTION <36hr AGO? —YES→ CHECK PARACETAMOL LEVELS

CHECK PARACETAMOL LEVELS AT 4hrs

NO ↓

PARACETAMOL LEVELS IN 'TOXIC' RANGE? (see graph below) —NO→

YES ↓

MONITOR:
• Liver function tests
• Prothrombin time
• Glucose
• Urea and Electrolytes

TREAT WITH N-ACETYLCYSTEINE
150mg/kg I/V over 15min
50mg/kg I/V over 4hr in 500ml 5% glucose
50mg/kg I/V over 8hr in 500ml 5% glucose
50mg/kg I/V over 8hr in 500ml 5% glucose

HEPATIC FAILURE WITH ENCEPHALOPATHY? —YES→

☎ EARLY REFERRAL TO HEPATOLOGIST

OBSERVE. COMPLICATIONS UNLIKELY

NO ↓

FULMINANT HEPATIC FAILURE ALGORITHM

OLIGURIA or RENAL FAILURE? —YES→

NO ↓

AVOID HYPOVOLAEMIA
OLIGURIA ALGORITHM
EARLY HAEMODIALYSIS

GRAPH FOR PREDICTION OF N-ACETYLCYSTEINE REQUIREMENT

TREATMENT WITH N-ACETYLCYSTEINE REQUIRED

TREATMENT WITH N-ACETYLCYSTEINE NOT REQUIRED

Paracetamol level (mmol/l)

Time since ingestion (hr)

PROLONGED PROTHROMBIN TIME? —YES→ VITAMIN K 10mg I/V od

NO ↓

RAISED BILIRUBIN? —YES→ ☎ EARLY REFERRAL TO HEPATOLOGIST

GENERAL SUPPORTIVE CARE
• Respiration
• Circulation
• Nutrition

NO ↓

HYPOGLYCAEMIA? —NO→

YES ↓

GLUCOSE 25g I/V prn
CONSIDER 10% GLUCOSE INFUSION

151

9.3 Salicylate poisoning

Toxicity of salicylate
1. Serious, life-threatening toxicity is likely after ingestion of >7.5 g salicylate.
2. In addition to aspirin poisoning salicylic acid (used as a keratolytic) or methylsalicylate (oil of wintergreen) may cause poisoning.
3. Salicylate is rapidly absorbed from the stomach and upper small bowel. Normal metabolic pathways are rapidly saturated requiring pH dependent renal elimination.
4. Toxicity is associated with complex metabolic derangement:
   - respiratory alkalosis due to stimulation of the respiratory centre
   - dehydration due to salt and water depletion associated with renal bicarbonate loss and hyperthermia
   - hypokalaemia associated with renal bicarbonate loss
   - metabolic acidosis due to interference with carbohydrate, lipid and amino acid metabolism
   - hyperthermia due to uncoupling of oxidative phosphorylation with wastage of energy as heat and increased metabolic rate
5. Salicylate poisoning may be complicated by capillary leak leading to pulmonary oedema.
6. Serious toxicity is associated with salicylate levels > 3.1 mmol/l. Above 6.2 mmol/l toxicity is life-threatening and respiratory depression may occur.
7. Continued absorption may cause levels to rise; repeated samples are therefore necessary.
8. Tissue binding of salicylate may lead to underestimation of severity of poisoning if levels are not taken before 12 hr after ingestion.
9. Salicylate reduces prothrombin levels but G-I bleeding and erosions are uncommon in acute toxicity.

Elimination of salicylate via bowel
1. Due to delayed gastric emptying induced emesis or gastric lavage may be useful up to 24 hr.
2. Activated charcoal should be used in repeated doses:
   - to adsorb salicylate remaining in the bowel
   - to adsorb salicylate back diffusing across the bowel mucosa

Alkaline diuresis
1. Alkalinization of the urine is necessary to increase renal elimination of salicylate.
2. Increased urinary alkali excretion is associated with hypokalaemia; careful monitoring and replacement of potassium is necessary.
3. Urinary alkalinization is more important for salicylate excretion than a diuresis.
4. A urine output >100 ml/hr should be maintained; frusemide or mannitol, in addition to intravenous crystalloids, may be necessary to achieve this.
5. Arterial pH should not be allowed to increase above 7.5. Bicarbonate infusion should be stopped if the arterial pH is high.
6. If urine fails to alkalinize with bicarbonate infusion further potassium repletion will be required.
7. Alkaline diuresis should be continued until serum salicylate levels are <3.1 mmol/l.
8. If alkaline diuresis continues for longer than 6 hr 10 ml 10% calcium gluconate should be given 6 hrly.

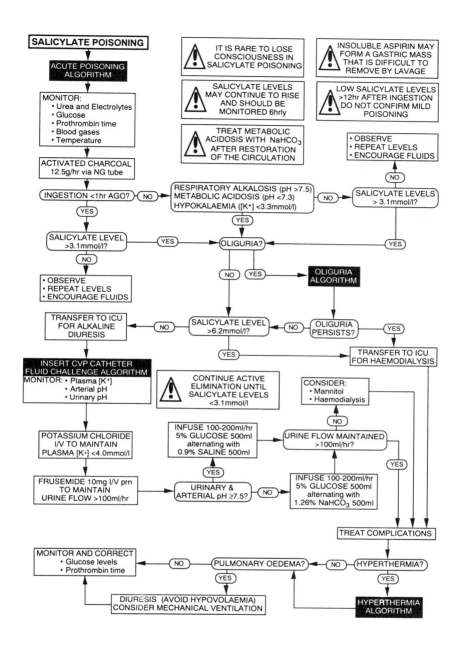

Bibliography

Hormaechea E, Carlson RW, Rogrove H, *et al.* Hypovolaemia, pulmonary oedema and protein changes in severe salicylate poisoning. *Am J Med* 1979; **66**:1046

Krause DS, Wolf BA, Shaw LM. Acute aspirin overdose: mechanisms of toxicity. *Ther Drug Monit* 1992; **14**:441

Notarianni L. A reassessment of the treatment of salicylate poisoning. *Drug Saf* 1992; **7**:292

Temple AR. Acute and chronic affects of aspirin toxicity and their treatment. *Arch Intern Med* 1981; **141**:364

10. Miscellaneous

10.1 Acute confusional state

Causes

1. Numerous causes exist, the commonest being related to drugs (or drug/alcohol withdrawal), infection, respiratory failure, metabolic causes (especially hypoglycaemia), head trauma and cerebral hypoperfusion (e.g. severe heart failure).
2. A careful history, examination and appropriate investigations should be performed.
3. Consider subdural haematoma if a recent history of head injury is obtained. A fluctuating level of consciousness or confusion need not be present.
4. Alcohol withdrawal symptoms generally occur 2–5 days after stopping intake.
5. Hypoglycaemia often occurs in conjunction with alcoholic intoxication.
6. Meningo-encephalitis may present as an acute confusional state.

Management

1. Treat the cause wherever possible rather than symptoms alone.
2. Confusion should *not* be treated with intravenous sedative agents (e.g. chlormethiazole, diazepam) unless the patient is in a carefully supervised, well-monitored area. Pulse oximetry provides a false sense of security as severe hypercapnia may occur before hypoxaemia develops.
3. Hypoxaemia should always be corrected. If sedation is required to keep an oxygen mask correctly placed then small aliquots should be given to provide sedation without respiratory depression. The patient should be carefully supervised in a well-monitored area.
4. Major tranquilizers such as chlorpromazine (50–100 mg P/O or I/M) and haloperidol (5–10 mg P/O or I/M) may cause hypotension and respiratory depression if given in excessive dosage. If possible, wait 20 minutes before administering a further dose.
5. Ensure patient safety, e.g. bedside rails.

Bibliography

Petersen RC. Acute confusional state. Don't mistake it for dementia. *Postgrad Med* 1992; **92**: 141
Tess MM. Acute confusional states in critically ill patients: a review. *J Neurosci Nurs* 1991; **23**: 398

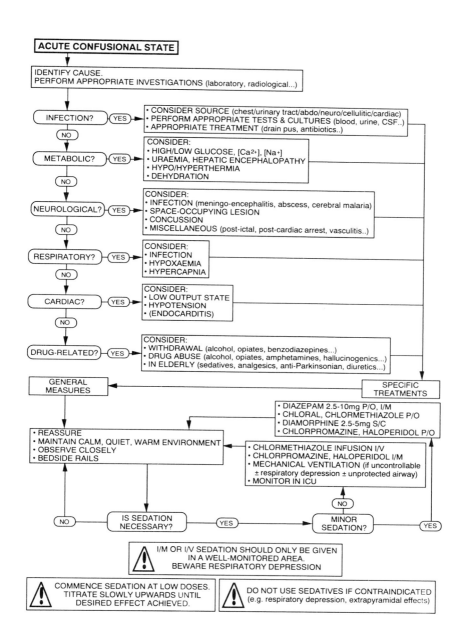

ACUTE CONFUSIONAL STATE

IDENTIFY CAUSE.
PERFORM APPROPRIATE INVESTIGATIONS (laboratory, radiological...)

INFECTION? — YES
- CONSIDER SOURCE (chest/urinary tract/abdo/neuro/cellulitic/cardiac)
- PERFORM APPROPRIATE TESTS & CULTURES (blood, urine, CSF..)
- APPROPRIATE TREATMENT (drain pus, antibiotics..)

NO

METABOLIC? — YES
CONSIDER:
- HIGH/LOW GLUCOSE, [Ca²⁺], [Na⁺]
- URAEMIA, HEPATIC ENCEPHALOPATHY
- HYPO/HYPERTHERMIA
- DEHYDRATION

NO

NEUROLOGICAL? — YES
CONSIDER:
- INFECTION (meningo-encephalitis, abscess, cerebral malaria)
- SPACE-OCCUPYING LESION
- CONCUSSION
- MISCELLANEOUS (post-ictal, post-cardiac arrest, vasculitis..)

NO

RESPIRATORY? — YES
CONSIDER:
- INFECTION
- HYPOXAEMIA
- HYPERCAPNIA

NO

CARDIAC? — YES
CONSIDER:
- LOW OUTPUT STATE
- HYPOTENSION
- (ENDOCARDITIS)

NO

DRUG-RELATED? — YES
CONSIDER:
- WITHDRAWAL (alcohol, opiates, benzodiazepines...)
- DRUG ABUSE (alcohol, opiates, amphetamines, hallucinogenics...)
- IN ELDERLY (sedatives, analgesics, anti-Parkinsonian, diuretics...)

GENERAL MEASURES

SPECIFIC TREATMENTS

- DIAZEPAM 2.5-10mg P/O, I/M
- CHLORAL, CHLORMETHIAZOLE P/O
- DIAMORPHINE 2.5-5mg S/C
- CHLORPROMAZINE, HALOPERIDOL P/O

- REASSURE
- MAINTAIN CALM, QUIET, WARM ENVIRONMENT
- OBSERVE CLOSELY
- BEDSIDE RAILS

- CHLORMETHIAZOLE INFUSION I/V
- CHLORPROMAZINE, HALOPERIDOL I/M
- MECHANICAL VENTILATION (if uncontrollable
  ± respiratory depression ± unprotected airway)
- MONITOR IN ICU

NO

NO — IS SEDATION NECESSARY? — YES — MINOR SEDATION? — YES

⚠ I/M OR I/V SEDATION SHOULD ONLY BE GIVEN
IN A WELL-MONITORED AREA.
BEWARE RESPIRATORY DEPRESSION

⚠ COMMENCE SEDATION AT LOW DOSES.
TITRATE SLOWLY UPWARDS UNTIL
DESIRED EFFECT ACHIEVED.

⚠ DO NOT USE SEDATIVES IF CONTRAINDICATED
(e.g. respiratory depression, extrapyramidal effects)

10.2 Acute anaemia

1. A drop in haemoglobin will result in a fall in tissue oxygen delivery (= Hb × cardiac output × arterial oxygen saturation × 1.34). Excessive falls in oxygen delivery will result in an inability to meet tissue oxygen demands leading to anaerobic metabolism and development of a lactic acidosis.
2. Chronic anaemia will be compensated for by an increase in cardiac output. The cardiac output often increases by 50–100% in patients with sickle cell disease.
3. Haemolysis is suggested by a reticulocytosis, a macrocytosis and an uncongugated hyperbilirubinaemia. The Coombs test will be positive with immune causes (may be drug-related).
4. A microcytic picture is commonly due to iron deficiency; thalassaemia should also be considered.
5. A normocytic picture is seen in anaemias of chronic disease, bone marrow failure, haemolysis, renal failure, pregnancy and hypothyroidism.
6. A macrocytic picture is often associated with vitamin B12 or folate deficiency, as well as chronic alcoholism, liver disease, myelodysplastic states and hypothyroidism.
7. Causes of haemolysis include:
   * malaria
   * drugs (e.g. high dose penicillin, methyldopa)
   * sickle cell crisis
   * thalassaemia
   * G6PD deficiency
   * hypersplenism
   * immune (Rhesus, warm or cold Ab)
   * haemolytic uraemic syndrome
   * cardiac valve prosthesis

Sickle cell crisis

1. Anaemia may be due to haemolytic, aplastic or sequestration crises.
2. A specialist haematological opinion should be sought urgently.

Treatment

1. Rapid blood transfusion may precipitate pulmonary oedema if given to euvolaemic or hypervolaemic patients, particularly the elderly. Monitoring is essential in these patients and small boluses of frusemide may be required with each bag of blood (preferably packed RBC).
2. For acute severe anaemias the haemoglobin should be elevated to 10 g/dl; however, in chronic anaemic states restoration to 8 g/dl may be sufficient.
3. For acutely ill patients with a megaloblastic anaemia, both B12 and folate should be given before laboratory results are known as folate alone may result in subacute combined degeneration of the spinal cord.

Bibliography

Massey AC. Microcytic anemia. Differential diagnosis and management of iron deficiency anemia. *Med Clin North Am* 1992; **76**: 549

Miller WM. Anemia in women ages 20 to 89 years; rationale and tools for differential diagnosis. *Clin Ther* 1993; **15**: 192

Rockey DC, Cello JP. Evaluation of the gastrointestinal tract in patients with iron-deficiency anemia. *N Engl J Med* 1993; **329**: 1691

Steingart R. Management of patients with sickle cell disease. *Med Clin North Am* 1992; **76**: 669

Tabbara IA. Hemolytic anemias. Diagnosis and management. *Med Clin North Am* 1992; **76**: 649

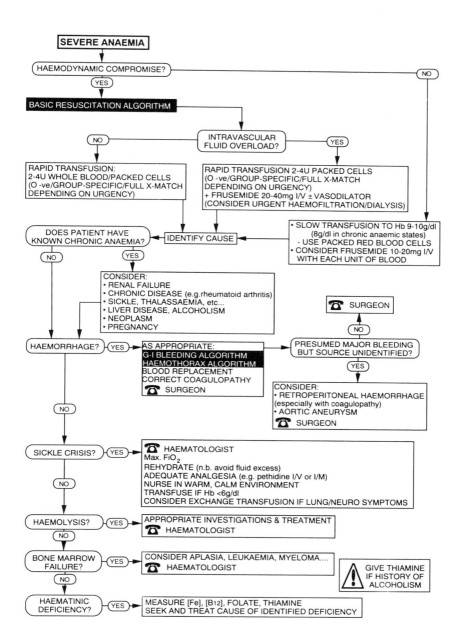

SEVERE ANAEMIA

HAEMODYNAMIC COMPROMISE? ──────────────────────────────── NO

YES

BASIC RESUSCITATION ALGORITHM

INTRAVASCULAR FLUID OVERLOAD?

NO

YES

RAPID TRANSFUSION:
2-4U WHOLE BLOOD/PACKED CELLS
(O -ve/GROUP-SPECIFIC/FULL X-MATCH
DEPENDING ON URGENCY)

RAPID TRANSFUSION 2-4U PACKED CELLS
(O -ve/GROUP-SPECIFIC/FULL X-MATCH
DEPENDING ON URGENCY)
+ FRUSEMIDE 20-40mg I/V ± VASODILATOR
(CONSIDER URGENT HAEMOFILTRATION/DIALYSIS)

IDENTIFY CAUSE

• SLOW TRANSFUSION TO Hb 9-10g/dl
  (8g/dl in chronic anaemic states)
  - USE PACKED RED BLOOD CELLS
• CONSIDER FRUSEMIDE 10-20mg I/V
  WITH EACH UNIT OF BLOOD

DOES PATIENT HAVE KNOWN CHRONIC ANAEMIA?

NO   YES

CONSIDER:
• RENAL FAILURE
• CHRONIC DISEASE (e.g.rheumatoid arthritis)
• SICKLE, THALASSAEMIA, etc...
• LIVER DISEASE, ALCOHOLISM
• NEOPLASM
• PREGNANCY

☎ SURGEON

NO

HAEMORRHAGE? — YES ─►

AS APPROPRIATE:
G-I BLEEDING ALGORITHM
HAEMOTHORAX ALGORITHM
BLOOD REPLACEMENT
CORRECT COAGULOPATHY
☎ SURGEON

PRESUMED MAJOR BLEEDING BUT SOURCE UNIDENTIFIED?

YES

CONSIDER:
• RETROPERITONEAL HAEMORRHAGE
(especially with coagulopathy)
• AORTIC ANEURYSM
☎ SURGEON

NO

SICKLE CRISIS? — YES ─►

☎ HAEMATOLOGIST
Max. FiO$_2$
REHYDRATE (n.b. avoid fluid excess)
ADEQUATE ANALGESIA (e.g. pethidine I/V or I/M)
NURSE IN WARM, CALM ENVIRONMENT
TRANSFUSE IF Hb <6g/dl
CONSIDER EXCHANGE TRANSFUSION IF LUNG/NEURO SYMPTOMS

NO

HAEMOLYSIS? — YES ─►

APPROPRIATE INVESTIGATIONS & TREATMENT
☎ HAEMATOLOGIST

NO

BONE MARROW FAILURE? — YES ─►

CONSIDER APLASIA, LEUKAEMIA, MYELOMA....
☎ HAEMATOLOGIST

⚠ GIVE THIAMINE IF HISTORY OF ALCOHOLISM

NO

HAEMATINIC DEFICIENCY? — YES ─►

MEASURE [Fe], [B12], FOLATE, THIAMINE
SEEK AND TREAT CAUSE OF IDENTIFIED DEFICIENCY

10.3 Pyrexia

History

1. A careful history should be taken, including recent travel, contacts (human and animal), and recent surgery.
2. One study revealed infection to be responsible for 27% of all pyrexias, multi-system diseases for 22%, tumours for 7%, drug fever for 3%, miscellaneous 14%, and no cause was isolated in 25%.

Infection

1. Infection should be excluded before other causes of pyrexia are entertained.
2. Pus should be actively sought and drained, especially when the pyrexia is swinging.
3. Nosocomial (hospital-acquired) infections are frequently related to (i) urinary and vascular catheters or cannulae, (ii) wounds, (iii) decreased chest movements and immobility. Gram negative organisms, often multiply-resistant to antibiotics, are more common causative agents.
4. If a cannula or catheter infection is suspected yet the patient is not systemically unwell, removal of the cannula/catheter may be sufficient without necessarily commencing antibiotics.
5. Strict aseptic technique should be used for all catheter and cannula insertions and manipulations.
6. As many specimens as appropriate should be taken for culture before commencement of antibiotic therapy.
7. Immunocompromised patients should receive antibiotic therapy if febrile.
8. Consider specific infections e.g. malaria, TB, Legionnaire's disease.
9. In the elderly, infection may present with subnormal temperatures.
10. Antibiotic courses should not be given for longer than necessary.

Other causes

1. If a transfusion reaction to blood products is suspected, stop the transfusion immediately and seek advice from the laboratory. The bag with the remaining blood products should be retained for subsequent analysis.
2. Very hot weather, or excessive temperature settings on an air-fluidized bed may cause non-swinging pyrexias.
3. If a cause for the pyrexia is not found, consider bacterial endocarditis, TB, sinusitis, and neoplasm (particularly lymphoma and renal cell carcinoma).
4. If multisystem symptoms and signs are present, consider connective tissue diseases.
5. Antibiotics and other drugs may be responsible for unexplained pyrexias. If possible, stop therapy and observe. Reculture after 24 hrs.

Treatment

1. Cooling measures (e.g. paracetamol, tepid sponging...) should be instituted for symptomatic relief.
2. Reduction of pyrexia may also improve haemodynamic stability.
3. Fans should not be directed directly at the patient but rather should aim to circulate air currents so that the patient loses more heat through convective losses.
4. Direct cooling of the skin with *cold* water, etc. results in peripheral vasoconstriction thereby not allowing the core temperature to dissipate.
5. Tepid sponging/wet sheets result in heat losses by the latent heat of evaporation.

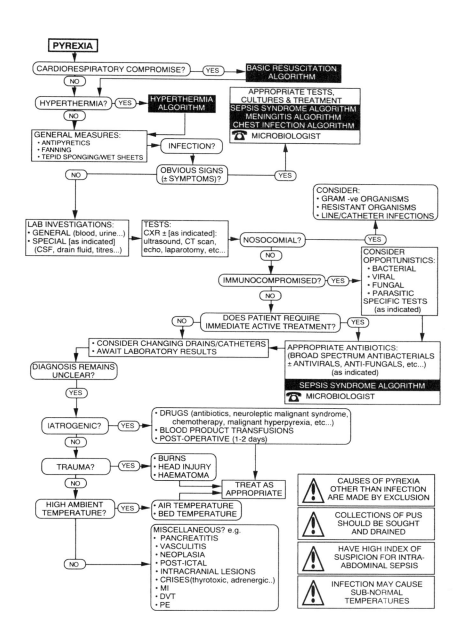

PYREXIA

CARDIORESPIRATORY COMPROMISE? — YES → **BASIC RESUSCITATION ALGORITHM**

NO

HYPERTHERMIA? — YES → **HYPERTHERMIA ALGORITHM**

NO

GENERAL MEASURES:
• ANTIPYRETICS
• FANNING
• TEPID SPONGING/WET SHEETS

→ INFECTION?

APPROPRIATE TESTS, CULTURES & TREATMENT
SEPSIS SYNDROME ALGORITHM
MENINGITIS ALGORITHM
CHEST INFECTION ALGORITHM
☎ MICROBIOLOGIST

OBVIOUS SIGNS (± SYMPTOMS)? — YES →

NO

CONSIDER:
• GRAM -ve ORGANISMS
• RESISTANT ORGANISMS
• LINE/CATHETER INFECTIONS

LAB INVESTIGATIONS:
• GENERAL (blood, urine...)
• SPECIAL [as indicated] (CSF, drain fluid, titres...)

TESTS:
CXR ± [as indicated]: ultrasound, CT scan, echo, laparotomy, etc...

NOSOCOMIAL? — YES →

NO

IMMUNOCOMPROMISED? — YES →

CONSIDER OPPORTUNISTICS:
• BACTERIAL
• VIRAL
• FUNGAL
• PARASITIC
SPECIFIC TESTS (as indicated)

NO

NO ← DOES PATIENT REQUIRE IMMEDIATE ACTIVE TREATMENT? — YES →

• CONSIDER CHANGING DRAINS/CATHETERS
• AWAIT LABORATORY RESULTS

APPROPRIATE ANTIBIOTICS:
(BROAD SPECTRUM ANTIBACTERIALS ± ANTIVIRALS, ANTI-FUNGALS, etc...) (as indicated)
SEPSIS SYNDROME ALGORITHM
☎ MICROBIOLOGIST

DIAGNOSIS REMAINS UNCLEAR?

YES

IATROGENIC? — YES →

• DRUGS (antibiotics, neuroleptic malignant syndrome, chemotherapy, malignant hyperpyrexia, etc...)
• BLOOD PRODUCT TRANSFUSIONS
• POST-OPERATIVE (1-2 days)

NO

TRAUMA? — YES →
• BURNS
• HEAD INJURY
• HAEMATOMA

NO

TREAT AS APPROPRIATE

HIGH AMBIENT TEMPERATURE? — YES →
• AIR TEMPERATURE
• BED TEMPERATURE

NO →

MISCELLANEOUS? e.g.
• PANCREATITIS
• VASCULITIS
• NEOPLASIA
• POST-ICTAL
• INTRACRANIAL LESIONS
• CRISES(thyrotoxic, adrenergic..)
• MI
• DVT
• PE

⚠ CAUSES OF PYREXIA OTHER THAN INFECTION ARE MADE BY EXCLUSION

⚠ COLLECTIONS OF PUS SHOULD BE SOUGHT AND DRAINED

⚠ HAVE HIGH INDEX OF SUSPICION FOR INTRA-ABDOMINAL SEPSIS

⚠ INFECTION MAY CAUSE SUB-NORMAL TEMPERATURES

Bibliography

Barbado FJ, Vazquez JJ, Pena JM, Arnalich F, Ortiz-Vazquez J. Pyrexia of unknown origin: changing spectrum of diseases in two consecutive series. *Postgrad Med J* 1992; **68**: 884

Berland B, Gleckman RA. Fever of unknown origin in the elderly. A sequential approach to diagnosis. *Postgrad Med* 1992; **92**: 197

Knockaert DC, Vanneste LJ, Vanneste SB, Bobbaers HJ. Fever of unknown origin in the 1980s. An update of the diagnostic spectrum. *Arch Intern Med* 1992; **152**: 51

Knockaert DC, Vanneste LJ, Bobbaers HJ. Recurrent or episodic fever of unknown origin. Review of 45 cases and survey of the literature. *Medicine Baltimore* 1993; **72**: 184

Molyneux M, Fox R. Diagnosis and treatment of malaria in Britain. *BMJ* 1993; **306**: 1175

Petersdorf RG. Fever of unknown origin. An old friend revisted. *Arch Intern Med* 1992; **152**: 21

Notes

10.4 Sepsis syndrome

1. Sepsis syndrome is an uncontrolled host inflammatory response to infection or tissue damage.
2. Control of the sepsis syndrome requires early and aggressive removal of the source:
   - drainage of pus
   - broad spectrum parenteral antibiotic therapy
   - aggressive debridement of all unclean wounds
   - early fixation of fractures

Physiological defects in the sepsis syndrome

1. Septicaemic shock is associated with failure of all components of the circulation
   - relative hypovolaemia
   - cardiac dysfunction
   - peripheral vascular failure
2. Peripheral vascular failure and right ventricular failure are significant factors in mortality.
4. Organ failure is associated with anaerobic metabolism and lactate production.
5. Lactaemia may also be due to impaired hepatic clearance.

Volume therapy

1. Due to capillary leak, intravascular volume expansion is often required despite oedema.
2. Stroke volume should usually be maximized with colloid before starting inotropes.
3. The stroke volume response to increases in filling pressure is depressed in septic shock.

Inotrope and vasopressor therapy

1. Severe shock may require inotropic and vasopressor support after correction of hypovolaemia.
2. Patient requiring catecholamine support should be invasively monitored in the ICU.
3. Catecholamine resistance may require high dosages of inotropes and vasopressors.
4. Vasopressors may increase filling pressures thus masking hypovolaemia.
5. Vasopressors may reduce cardiac output and therefore tissue oxygen delivery.
6. If cardiac output requires inotropic support this should be started before using vasopressors.
7. The smallest dose of vasopressor should be used to obtain an acceptable mean arterial pressure.

Bibliography

Balk RA, Parrillo JE. Prognostic factors in sepsis: the cold facts. *Crit Care Med* 1992; **20**:1373

Bone RC, Fisher CJ, Clemmer TP, *et al.* The sepsis syndrome: a valid clinical entity. *Crit Care Med* 1989; **17**:389

Edwards JD, Brown CS, Nightingale P, *et al.* Use of survivors' cardio-respiratory values as therapeutic goals in septic shock. *Crit Care Med* 1989; **17**:1098

Ellman H. Capillary permeability in septic patients. *Crit Care Med* 1984; **12**:629

Groenveld ABJ, Bronsveld W, Thijs LG. Hemodynamic determinants of mortality in human septic shock. *Surgery* 1986; **99**:140

Imm A, Carlson RW. Fluid resuscitation in circulatory shock. *Crit Care Clin* 1993; **9**:313

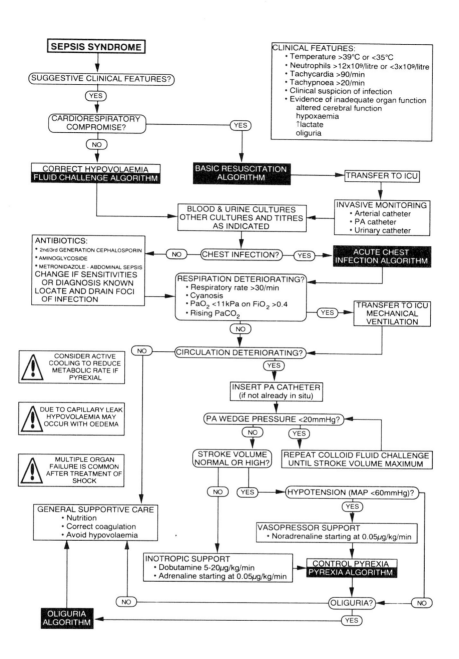

SEPSIS SYNDROME

SUGGESTIVE CLINICAL FEATURES?
→ YES

CLINICAL FEATURES:
• Temperature >39°C or <35°C
• Neutrophils >12x10⁹/litre or <3x10⁹/litre
• Tachycardia >90/min
• Tachypnoea >20/min
• Clinical suspicion of infection
• Evidence of inadequate organ function
   altered cerebral function
   hypoxaemia
   ↑lactate
   oliguria

CARDIORESPIRATORY COMPROMISE?
→ YES → BASIC RESUSCITATION ALGORITHM → TRANSFER TO ICU
→ NO

CORRECT HYPOVOLAEMIA
FLUID CHALLENGE ALGORITHM

INVASIVE MONITORING
• Arterial catheter
• PA catheter
• Urinary catheter

BLOOD & URINE CULTURES
OTHER CULTURES AND TITRES
AS INDICATED

ANTIBIOTICS:
• 2nd/3rd GENERATION CEPHALOSPORIN
• AMINOGLYCOSIDE
• METRONIDAZOLE - ABDOMINAL SEPSIS
CHANGE IF SENSITIVITIES
OR DIAGNOSIS KNOWN
LOCATE AND DRAIN FOCI
OF INFECTION

NO ← CHEST INFECTION? → YES → **ACUTE CHEST INFECTION ALGORITHM**

RESPIRATION DETERIORATING?
• Respiratory rate >30/min
• Cyanosis
• PaO₂ <11kPa on FiO₂ >0.4
• Rising PaCO₂
→ YES → TRANSFER TO ICU MECHANICAL VENTILATION
→ NO

⚠ CONSIDER ACTIVE COOLING TO REDUCE METABOLIC RATE IF PYREXIAL

NO ← CIRCULATION DETERIORATING?
→ YES

⚠ DUE TO CAPILLARY LEAK HYPOVOLAEMIA MAY OCCUR WITH OEDEMA

INSERT PA CATHETER
(if not already in situ)

PA WEDGE PRESSURE <20mmHg?
→ NO / → YES

⚠ MULTIPLE ORGAN FAILURE IS COMMON AFTER TREATMENT OF SHOCK

STROKE VOLUME NORMAL OR HIGH?
REPEAT COLLOID FLUID CHALLENGE UNTIL STROKE VOLUME MAXIMUM

GENERAL SUPPORTIVE CARE
• Nutrition
• Correct coagulation
• Avoid hypovolaemia

→ NO / → YES → HYPOTENSION (MAP <60mmHg)?
→ YES

VASOPRESSOR SUPPORT
• Noradrenaline starting at 0.05µg/kg/min

INOTROPIC SUPPORT
• Dobutamine 5-20µg/kg/min
• Adrenaline starting at 0.05µg/kg/min
→ **CONTROL PYREXIA PYREXIA ALGORITHM**

NO ← OLIGURIA? ← NO

OLIGURIA ALGORITHM
← YES

Meadows D, Edwards JD, Wilkins RG, *et al*. Reversal of intractable septic shock with nor-epinephrine therapy. *Crit Care Med* 1988; **16**:663

Ognibene FP, Parker MM, Natanson C, *et al*. Depressed left ventricular performance in response to volume infusion in patients with sepsis and septic shock. *Chest* 1988; **93**:903

Parker MM, Shelhamer JH, Bacharach SL, *et al*. Profound but reversible myocardial depression in patients with septic shock. *Ann Intern Med* 1984; **100**:483

Vincent JL, Bihari D. Sepsis, severe sepsis or sepsis syndrome: need for clarification. *Intensive Care Med* 1992; **18**:255

Welbourn CR, Young Y. Endotoxin, septic shock and acute lung injury: neutrophils, macrophages and inflammatory mediators. *Br J Surg* 1992; **79**:998

Wolf YG, Cotev S, Perel A, *et al*. Dependence of oxygen consumption on cardiac output in sepsis. *Crit Care Med* 1987; **15**:198

Notes

10.5 Anaphylactoid reaction

1. Many patients will have had a minor reaction to an allergen before a severe anaphylactoid reaction occurs; any history of reactions should be taken seriously.
2. Anaphylactoid reactions range from minor (itching, urticaria) to fatal with circulatory collapse and severe bronchospasm.
3. Most reactions are acute in onset and are clearly temporally related to the causative allergen; some complement mediated reactions may take longer to develop.
4. Reactions to long-acting drugs may be prolonged.

Clinical features

1. Respiratory disturbance includes laryngeal oedema, bronchospasm, pulmonary oedema due to capillary leak and pulmonary hypertension due to vascular occlusion.
2. Cardiovascular collapse may be due to massive capillary leak, peripheral vasodilatation and myocardial depression.
3. Which feature predominates depends on the immune mechanism underlying the reaction.

Treatment

1. Fluid replacement should be with colloid solutions and may require very large volumes to replace plasma volume deficit.
2. Military anti-shock trousers (MAST) may be considered acutely to divert blood centrally and to increase peripheral resistance.
3. Hydroxyethyl starch solutions are ideal for fluid replacement unless the reaction is considered to be due to hydroxyethyl starch (rare).
4. Plasma volume replacement is not adequate whilst the haemoglobin is high; a high haemoglobin underestimates the plasma volume deficit.
5. Adrenaline is the mainstay of drug treatment for bronchospasm and circulatory collapse.
6. Steroids are useful in prolonged reactions to suppress further deterioration. Although steroids are commonly given acutely they probably have little benefit in the short term.
7. Antihistamines are useful for urticaria and probably in prolonged shock.

Bibliography

Bickell WH, Dice WH. Military antishock trousers in a patient with adrenergic resistant anaphylaxis. *Ann Emerg Med* 1984; **13**:189

Fisher MM. Blood volume replacement in acute anaphylactic cardiovascular collapse. *Br J Anaesth* 1977; **49**:1023

Fisher MM. Clinical observations on the pathophysiology and treatment of anaphylactic cardiovascular collapse. *Anesth Intensive Care* 1986; **14**:17

Fisher MM. Treating anaphylaxis with sympathomimetic drugs. *BMJ* 1992; **305**:1107

Hollingsworth HM, Giansiracusa DF, Upchurch KS. Anaphylaxis. *J Intensive Care Med* 1991; **6**:55

Raper RR, Fisher MM. Profound reversible myocardial dysfunction after anaphylaxis. *Lancet* 1988; i:386

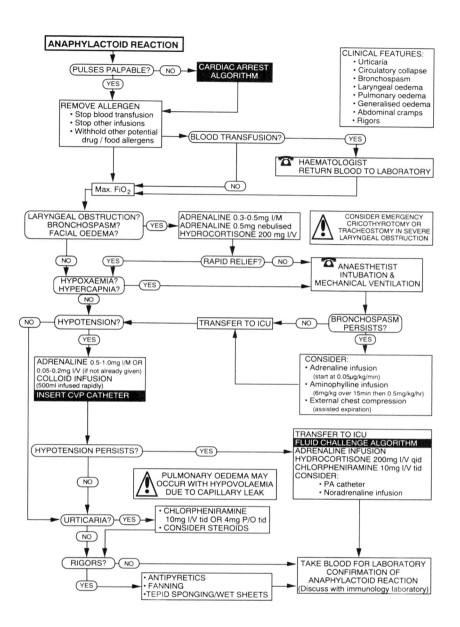

ANAPHYLACTOID REACTION

PULSES PALPABLE? —NO→ CARDIAC ARREST ALGORITHM

YES

CLINICAL FEATURES:
- Urticaria
- Circulatory collapse
- Bronchospasm
- Laryngeal oedema
- Pulmonary oedema
- Generalised oedema
- Abdominal cramps
- Rigors

REMOVE ALLERGEN
- Stop blood transfusion
- Stop other infusions
- Withhold other potential drug / food allergens

BLOOD TRANSFUSION? —YES→

☎ HAEMATOLOGIST RETURN BLOOD TO LABORATORY

NO

Max. FiO$_2$

LARYNGEAL OBSTRUCTION? BRONCHOSPASM? FACIAL OEDEMA? —YES→ ADRENALINE 0.3-0.5mg I/M ADRENALINE 0.5mg nebulised HYDROCORTISONE 200 mg I/V

⚠ CONSIDER EMERGENCY CRICOTHYROTOMY OR TRACHEOSTOMY IN SEVERE LARYNGEAL OBSTRUCTION

NO / YES

RAPID RELIEF? —NO→

☎ ANAESTHETIST INTUBATION & MECHANICAL VENTILATION

HYPOXAEMIA? HYPERCAPNIA? —YES→

NO

HYPOTENSION? ←TRANSFER TO ICU← —NO— BRONCHOSPASM PERSISTS?

NO

YES

YES

ADRENALINE 0.5-1.0mg I/M OR 0.05-0.2mg I/V (if not already given) COLLOID INFUSION (500ml infused rapidly) INSERT CVP CATHETER

CONSIDER:
- Adrenaline infusion (start at 0.05µg/kg/min)
- Aminophylline infusion (6mg/kg over 15min then 0.5mg/kg/hr)
- External chest compression (assisted expiration)

TRANSFER TO ICU
FLUID CHALLENGE ALGORITHM
ADRENALINE INFUSION
HYDROCORTISONE 200mg I/V qid
CHLORPHENIRAMINE 10mg I/V tid
CONSIDER:
- PA catheter
- Noradrenaline infusion

HYPOTENSION PERSISTS? —YES→

⚠ PULMONARY OEDEMA MAY OCCUR WITH HYPOVOLAEMIA DUE TO CAPILLARY LEAK

NO

URTICARIA? —YES→
- CHLORPHENIRAMINE 10mg I/V tid OR 4mg P/O tid
- CONSIDER STEROIDS

NO

RIGORS? —NO→ TAKE BLOOD FOR LABORATORY CONFIRMATION OF ANAPHYLACTOID REACTION (Discuss with immunology laboratory)

YES
- ANTIPYRETICS
- FANNING
- TEPID SPONGING/WET SHEETS

Index

Main references to algorithms are in **bold type**.

N-acetylcysteine 150–1
acidosis
  metabolic 10–11, 26–8, 52–5, 66–8,
  78, **82–4**, 110–12, 152–3
  respiratory 10
Addisonian crisis, *see* hypoadrenalism
adenosine 42–5
ADH, *see* antidiuretic hormone
adrenaline **2**, 9, 15, 26–8, 30–2, 46–8,
  50–1, 162–4, 166–7
adult respiratory distress syndrome
  ARDS **12–13**, 163
agitation, *see* confusion
airflow limitation,
  acute on chronic 3, 10–11, 12–13, 15,
  16–17
airway obstruction 8–9, 13
alcoholism 110–12, 114–16, 122–3,
  154–5
alkaline diuresis 146–8, 152–3
alkalosis
  metabolic 84–5, 106–7, 110–12
  respiratory 72–3, 152–3
aminophylline 15
amiodarone 39–41, 42–5
ammonium chloride 84–5
anaemia 11, **156–7**
  iron deficiency 156–7
  megaloblastic 156–7
anaphylactoid reaction 9, 11, 15, 38,
  166–7
angina 36–7
angiodysplasia 100–1
angiography 38–41, 50–1, 100–1
angioplasty 38–41
angiotensin converting enzyme (ACE)
  inhibitors 46–8
antacids 100–1
antibiotics 15, 18–20, 52–5, 108–9,
  132–4, 140–1, 158–60
anticonvulsants 122–3
antidiuretic hormone 58–60
  inappropriate 62–4
antiemetics **106–7**
antihistamines 38, 166–7
aortic
  aneursym 36–7, 38
  coarctation 34–5,
  dissection 35

aprotonin 38
arrhythmias 3, 4, 30–2, 38–41, **42–5**,
  79, 92–3, 110–12, 118–19, 128–30,
  146–8
aspirin, – *see* salicylate
asthma 12–13, **14–15**
atenolol 39–41
atropine 26–8, 40, 42–4

β_2-agonist 14–15
β-blockade 35, 38–41, 92–3, 38
benzodiazepines 122–3, 154–5
bicarbonate, sodium **26–8**, 56–7, **82–4**,
  86–9, 146–8
bradycardia, *see* arrhythmias
brain stem death 129, **142–3**
bronchitis 18, 20

calcitonin 70–1
calcium chloride/gluconate 26–8, 42–5,
  66–8, 152–3
calcium resonium 66–8
captopril 46–8
carbimazole 92–3
cardiac arrest 3, **26–8**, 38–41
cardiac output 30–2, 46–8
cardiogenic shock, *see* heart failure
catheter
  central venous 4–5, 6–7, 38, 50–1,
  100–1
  infection 158–60
  pulmonary artery 6–7, 31–2, 38, 50–1
cerebral oedema 110–12, 124–6
cerebrospinal fluid 132–4
cerebrovascular accident 128–30
chest drain **22–5**
chest infection 18–20, 36–7, 86
chlormethiazole 122–3, 154–5
chlorpheniramine, *see* antihistamines
coagulopathy 4, 23–5, 74–6, 100–1
colitis
  ischaemic 104–5, 108–9
  ulcerative 108–9
coma 3, 62–4, 70–1, 78–80, 86–9, 90–1,
  114–16, 128–30, 146–8
compartment syndrome 56–7
confusion 154–5

continuous positive airways pressure (CPAP) 12, 14, 17, 18–19, 46–8
convulsions, *see* seizures
costochondritis 36–7, 39
creatine phosphokinase (CPK) 38–41, 56–7
creatinine 52–5, 56–7
cyanide 34

D-dimer 50–1
dantrolene 74–6
dDAVP 58–60, 98–9, 102–3
defibrillation 26–8
dexamethasone, *see* steroid therapy
diabetes insipidus 58–60, 98–9
diabetes mellitus, *see* hyperglycaemia
dialysis, *see* renal replacement
diamorphine 36–7, 39–41
diarrhoea 108–9
digoxin 42–5, 68, 146–8
diltiazem 39–41
diphosphonates 70–1
disseminated intravascular coagulation (DIC) 74–6
diuretics 39–41, **46–8,** 52–5, 56–7, 58–60, 62–4, 70–1, 110–12, 124–6
dobutamine 30–2, 46–8, 162–4
dopamine 30–2, 46–8, 52–5, 162–4
doxapram 16–17
dyspnoea 9, **10–11**, 13, 50–1

eclampsia 35
encephalopathy 110–12, 114–16, 120–1, 124–6, **132–4**
epiglottitis **8–9**

fasciotomy 56–7
fits, *see* seizures
fluid challenge 6–7, 46–8, 50–1, 100–1
fluid overload 46–8
flumazenil 146–8
frusemide 39–41, **46–8,** 52–5, 56–7, 58–60, 62–4, 70–1, 110–12, 124–6, 152–3

gastrointestinal bleeding 100–1, 102–3
Glasgow Coma Scale 114–16, 124–6
glomerulonephritis, *see* nephritis
glucagon 90–1
glucose 66–8, 86–9, 90–1
glyceryl trinitrate (GTN), *see* nitrates
Guillain–Barré syndrome 118–9

H_2-antagonists 38, 100–1, 102–3
haematuria 56–7
haemofiltration, *see* renal replacement
haemoglobinuria 56–7
haemolysis 56–7, 74–6, 156–7
haemolytic uraemic syndrome 55
haemorrhage 7, 156–7
  intracranial 114–16
  subarachnoid 114–16, 120–1, 128–30
  variceal 102–3
haemothorax 13, **22–5**
headache 99, **120–1,** 124–6
heart block 42–5
heart failure 3, 11, 13, 30–2, 38–41, 42–5, **46–8**, 92–3, 94–5
Heimlich manoeuvre 8–9
Heliox 8–9
heparin 38–41, 50–1, 87–8
hepatic failure 106–7, **110–12**, 146–8, 154–5
hepatitis 110–12
hydralazine 35
hydrocortisone, *see* steroid therapy
hypercalcaemia 70–1
hypercapnia 2, **12–13,** 14–15, 16–17, 18
hyperglycaemia 39–41, **86–9,** 106–7, 114–16
  ketoacidosis 86–8
  non–ketotic crisis 58–60, **86–9**
hyperkalaemia 26–8, 52–5, 56–7, **66–7,** 74, 96–7
hypernatraemia 58–60
hypertension 34–5, 120–1, 128–30
hyperthermia 74–6, 114–16, 122–3, 152
hyperthyroidism, *see* thyrotoxic crisis
hyperventilation 10–11, 72–3, 124–6
hypoadrenalism 62–4, 94–5, **96–7**
hypocalcaemia 26–8, 56–7, **72–3**
hypoglycaemia 90–1, 96–7, 110–12, 114–16, 122–3, 151
hypokalaemia 45, **66–8,** 106–7, 110–12
hypomagnesaemia 72–3
hyponatraemia 62–4, 106–7
hypopituitary crisis 98–9
hypotension 2–3, 30–2, 38–41, 46–8, 52–5, 72–3, 100–1
  postural 7
hypothermia 78–80, 94–5, 114–16
hypothyroidism, *see* myxoedema
hypovolaemia 6–7, 18, 30–2, 46–8, 52–5, 58–60, 162–4
hypoxaemia 2, 10–11, **12–13,** 14–15, 16–17, 18–20, 23–5, 44, 46–8, 110–12, 114–16, 154–5

infection 154–5, 158–60, 162–4
  abdominal 104–5
  chest 15, 17, **18–20**
insulin 66–8, **86–9**, 90–1
inflammatory bowel disease 108–9 *see
  also* colitis
intraaortic balloon pump 31–2, 40
ipratropium 14–15
isoprenaline 30–2, 40, 43–4
isosorbide dinitrate, *see* nitrates

labetalol 35
lactic acidosis **46–8**, 82–4, 162–4
lignocaine 26–8, 39–41
lung collapse 16

magnesium sulphate 39–41, 42–5,
  122–3, 140–1
malabsorption 108–9
malaria 56–7, 90–1, 124–6
malignant hyperthermia 74–6
mannitol 52–5, 56–7, 124–6, 152–3
mechanical ventilation 2, 15, 16–17, 23,
  46–8, 50–1, 118–19, 124–6
meningitis 120–1, **132–4**
mixed venous oxygen saturation 46–8
myasthenia gravis 13, 118–19, **136–8**
myocardial infarction 36–7, **38–41**,
  44–5, 86
myoglobinuria 52–5, **56–7**
myxoedema 94–5, 96–7

naloxone 146–48
nephritis 35, 56–7
neuroleptic malignant syndrome 74–6
nifedipine 34–5, 39–41
nimodipine 128–30
nitrates 35, 39–41, 42–4, 46–8, 102–3
nitroprusside 34–5
non-steroidals 36–7, 39
noradrenaline 30–2, 162–4
nutrition 53–5, 106–7, 108–9, 110–12

oesophagitis 36–7
oliguria 46–8, **52–5**
opiates 36–7, 39–41
organ donation 144–5
osmolality 52–5, 98–9
oxygen therapy 10–11, 14–15, 16–17,
  18–19, 23–5

pacing 42–5
pain
  abdominal 70–1, 86, **104–5**
  chest 36–7, 50–1
  facial 120–1
  fictitious 104–5
pancreatitis 12, 70–1, 86, 104–5
papilloedema 35, 132–4
paracetamol poisoning 110–12, 146–8,
  150–1
peptic ulcer 36–7
pericardial tamponade 30–2, 48
pericarditis 36–7, 38–41
phaeochromocytoma 34–5
phenothiazines 154–5
phenytoin 122–3
plasma
  fresh frozen 38
plasmapheresis 118–19, 136–8
pleural effusion 5, 13, **22–5**
pleurisy 36–7, 50–1
pneumonia 18–20
pneumothorax 5, 13, 14–15, 16–17,
  22–5, 30–2, 36–7
poisoning 11, 13, 74–6, 106–7, 114–16,
  146–8
potassium chloride **66–8**
prednisolone, *see* steroid therapy
pre-eclampsia 35
pregnancy 35, 106–7
pressure
  central venous (CVP) **4–5, 6–7**, 46–8,
    162–4
  cerebral perfusion (CPP) 124–6
  intracranial (ICP) 35, 114–16, **124–6**
  pulmonary artery wedge (PAWP) 31,
    46–8, 162–4
  systemic 7, **30–2, 34–5**
propranolol 35, 39–41, 92–3
pulmonary embolus 13, 31, 36–7,
  50–1, 86–9
pulmonary oedema **46–8**
pyrexia 74–6, **158–60**; *see also* hyperthermia

ranitidine, *see* H$_2$-antagonists
renal
  failure 35, **52–5**, 72–3, 106–7,
    110–12, 154–5
  replacement 52–5, 56–7, 70–1
respiratory failure 11, **12–13**
resuscitation, cardiopulmonary 2, 15,
  20, 24–5, **26–8**, 38
rhabdomyolysis 52–5, **56–7**, 74–6

salbutamol 14–15
salicylate 11, 38–41, 74–6, 100–1, 128–30
  poisoning 152–3
sclerotherapy 102–3
sedatives 52–5, 140–1, 152–3
seizures 35, 62–4, **122–3**, 146–8
Seldinger technique 4
sepsis 110–12, 158–60, **162–4**
sickle cell crisis 56–7, 104–5, 156–7
sodium chloride 58–60, 62–4, 86–9, 96–7
steroid therapy 14–15, 38, 70–1, 92–3, 94–5, 96–7, 98–9, 120–1, 122–3, 124–6, 132–4, 136–8
streptokinase 38–41
stress ulceration 100–1
stridor 8–9
stroke, *see* cerebrovascular accident

tachyarrhythmia, *see* arrhythmia
temporal arteritis 128–30
tetanus 13, **140–1**
tetany 72–3
thirst 58–60
thrombocytopenia 74–6
thrombolysis 38–41, 50–1, 128–30
thyrotoxic crisis 92–3
thyroxine 94–5, 98–9

tissue plasminogen activator (rTPA) 38–41, 50–1
torsades de pointes 43–5
tracheostomy/tracheotomy 8–9, 166–7
tranexamic acid 38
transient ischaemic attack (TIA) 128
trauma 8–9, 12–13, 24–5, 36–7, 38, 158–60

unconsciousness, *see* coma
uraemia, *see* renal failure
urate nephropathy 55
urea 52–5, 56–7
urinalysis 52–5
urinary tract obstruction 52–5

variceal haemorrhage 100–1, **102–3**
vasculitis 35, 128–30
vasopressin, *see* dDAVP
verapamil 26–8, 42–5
vomiting 2, **106–7**

weakness 13, **118–19**
Waterhouse–Friedrichsen syndrome 96–7

X-ray, chest 4–5, 22–4, 37, 50–1